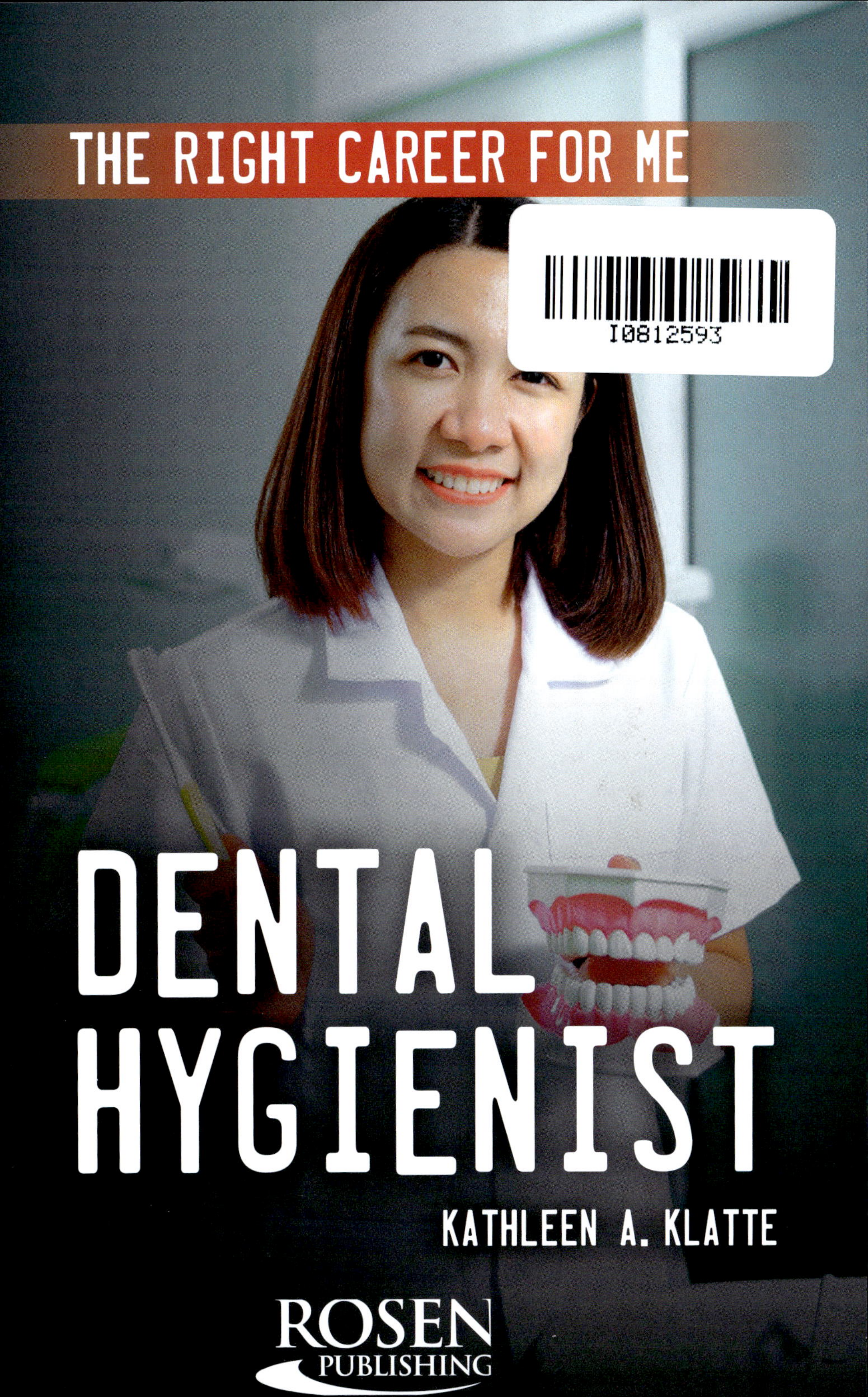

THE RIGHT CARER FOR ME

DENTAL HYGIENIST

KATHLEEN A. KLATTE

ROSEN PUBLISHING

Published in 2025 by The Rosen Publishing Group, Inc.
2544 Clinton Street, Buffalo, NY 14224

Cover Designer: Michael Flynn
Intertior Designer: Rachel Rising
Editor: Kathleen A. Klatte

Portions of this work were originally authored by Ann Byers and published as *A Career as a Dental Hygienist*. All new material in this edition was authored by Kathleen A. Klatte.

Cataloging-in-Publication Data

Names: Klatte, Kathleen A.
Title: Dental hygienist / Kathleen A. Klatte.
Description: Buffalo, NY : Rosen Publishing, 2025. | Series: The right career for me | Includes glossary and index.
Identifiers: ISBN 9781499476361 (pbk.) | ISBN 9781499476378 (library bound) | ISBN 9781499476385 (ebook)
Subjects: LCSH: Dental hygiene--Vocational guidance--Juvenile literature. | Dental hygienists--Juvenile literature.
Classification: LCC RK60.5 K525 2025 | DDC 617.6'0233--dc23

Manufactured in the United States of America

CPSIA Compliance Information: Batch #CSRYA25. For further information, contact Rosen Publishing at 1-800-237-9932.

CONTENTS

INTRODUCTION

Visiting the dentist is an essential part of health care. It's important to your overall heath and well-being to have a healthy mouth and teeth. There are different kinds of health care professionals who work in a dental clinic. A dentist is a medical doctor who specializes in caring for teeth, gums, and mouths. A dental assistant performs some of the duties of a receptionist such as organizing appointments and keeping records. They also take care of tasks such as cleaning the exam room between patients.

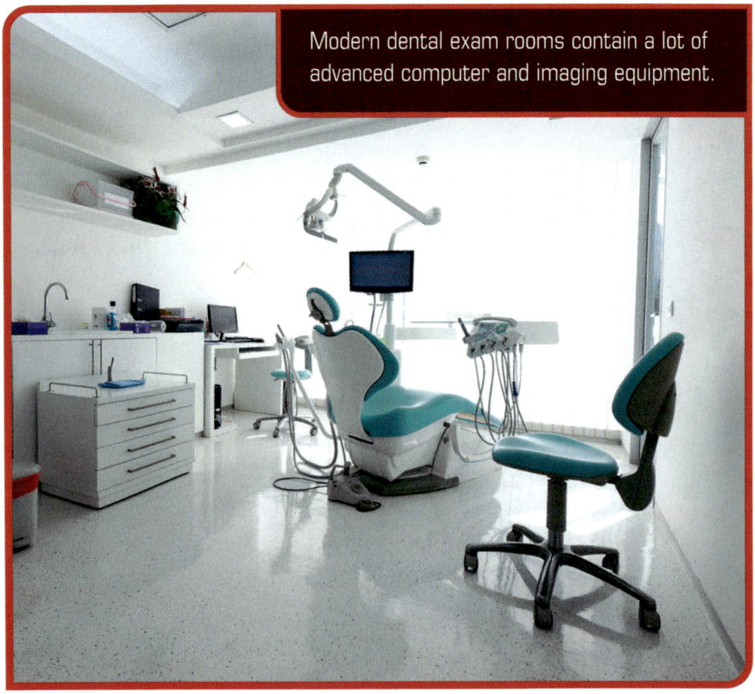

Modern dental exam rooms contain a lot of advanced computer and imaging equipment.

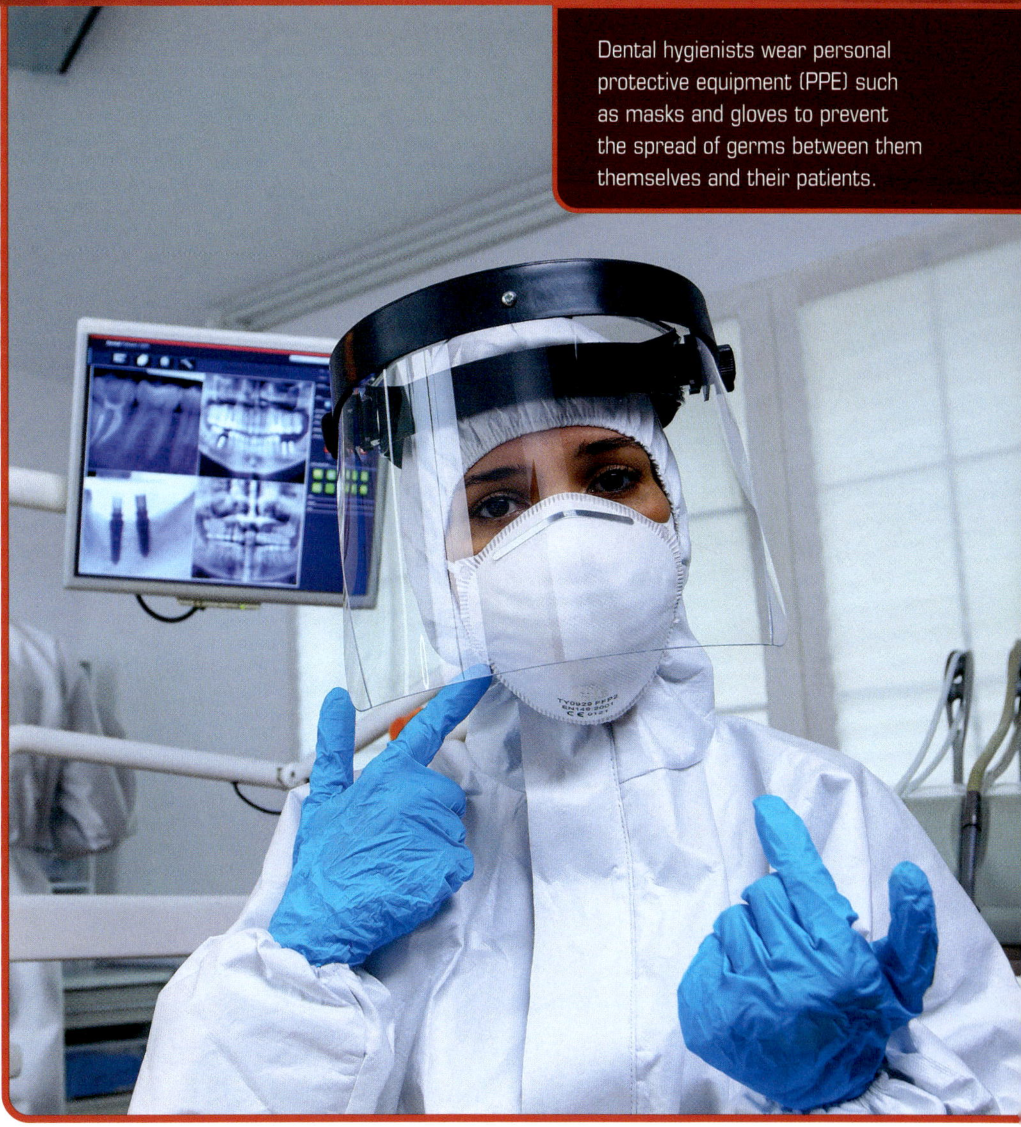

Dental hygienists wear personal protective equipment (PPE) such as masks and gloves to prevent the spread of germs between them themselves and their patients.

Perhaps the most flexible career option in dentistry is that of dental hygienist. Dental hygienists typically require an associate's degree and license to practice. Becoming a dental hygienist requires about three years of college—much less time and money than becoming a dentist, while still resulting in a challenging, well-paid career.

According to the U.S. Bureau of Labor Statistics (BLS) 93 percent of hygienists work in dental offices. The offices are usually very nice with top-quality, up-to-date equipment. A few practice in doctors' offices, health clinics, hospitals, and other health care settings. Some work in schools, in prisons, on military bases, or on Indian reservations. Hygienists work alongside dentists and dental assistants.

Hygienists can choose to work full-time or part-time, for one practice or several. They can often arrange their work hours to fit their scheduling needs. Another great benefit of a career as a dental hygienist is the fact that the job will always be needed.

MAKING A DIFFERENCE

Dental hygienist Judy Boothby recalls a particularly memorable patient. She'd been told the elderly woman was "difficult." She was always angry and seemed uncomfortable around people. She didn't want anyone poking around in her mouth. She probably recalled a time when it was common for dentists to berate their patients for the state of their teeth. But Boothby was not afraid of difficult patients. In her job as a dental hygienist, she worked mainly with older people. Most of her patients lived in nursing homes or assisted living apartments.

Even though the woman didn't want to see a dental hygienist, Boothby started visiting her. She found out why the woman stayed in her room all the time and why she was so unhappy. She didn't like the way she looked. She had only a few teeth, and several of them were broken. Others were decaying. She had dentures—false teeth—that didn't fit right.

She was embarrassed to open her mouth in front of people. Because her teeth were broken, she could not eat normal food; she had to have everything mashed up. In addition, the decay caused infections, bleeding, and pain. A dental hygienist was exactly what this miserable, lonely woman needed!

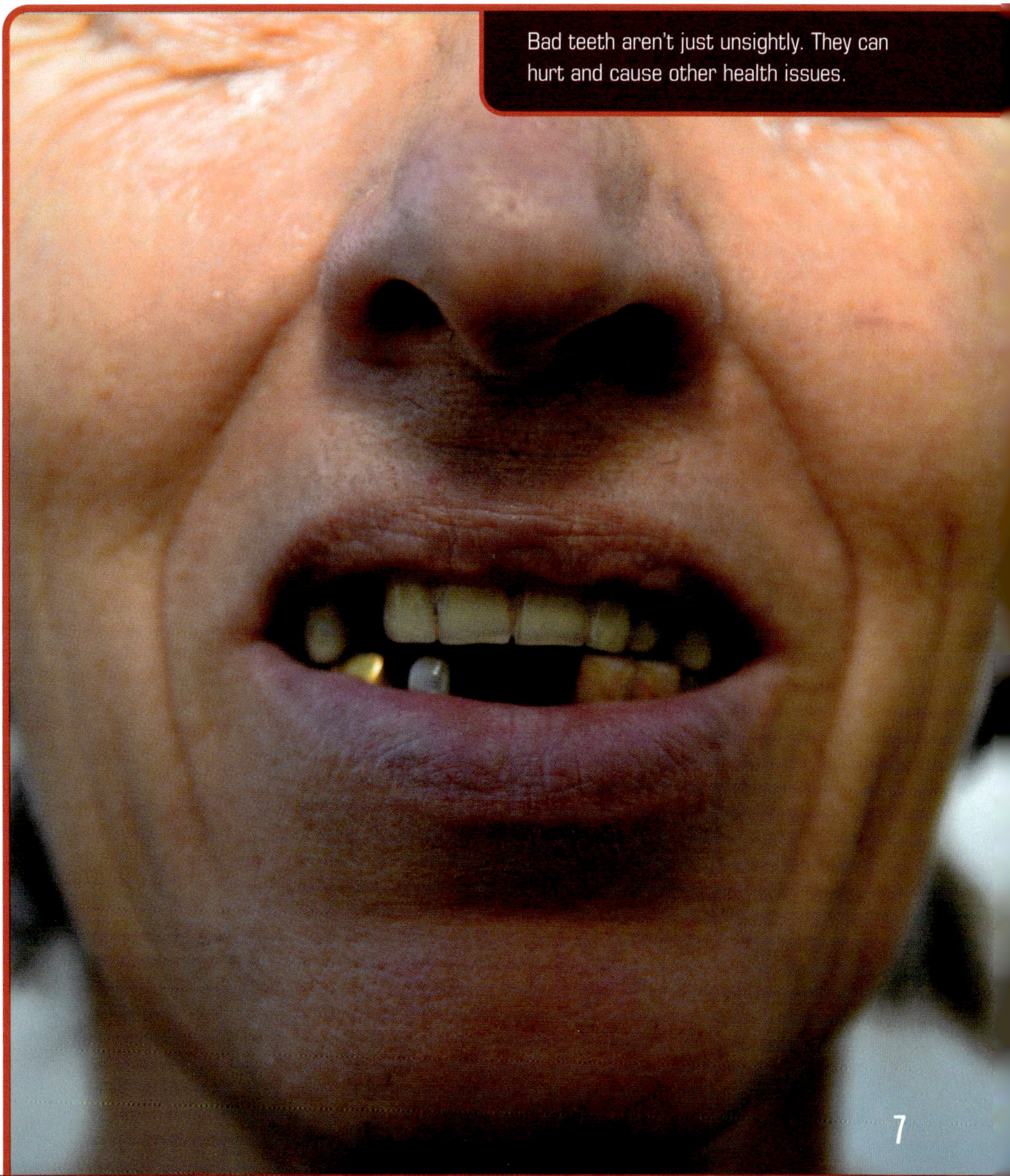

Bad teeth aren't just unsightly. They can hurt and cause other health issues.

Today, people who work in dentistry are trained to make their patients comfortable so they can address their medical issues without upsetting them. Boothby convinced the woman to let her help. She cleaned her teeth and got rid of the infection. She removed the decay and put temporary fillings in. She arranged for her to go to a dentist, who fixed the broken teeth and got her dentures to fit nicely.

These improvements in the woman's dental health brought huge changes in her life. She began going to the dining room and taking part in the home's activities. She talked and laughed with others. She ate better, so her overall health improved. She paid attention to her clothes and started wearing makeup. This difficult woman became a happy, friendly, and well-liked resident of her nursing home.

This woman's experience is one of the reasons why Boothby enjoys being a dental hygienist: she knows she is making a big difference in her patients' lives. She helps people correct problems and stay healthy. She spots small problems before they become big, and she refers her patients to dentists if they need treatment. She helps them feel and look their best.

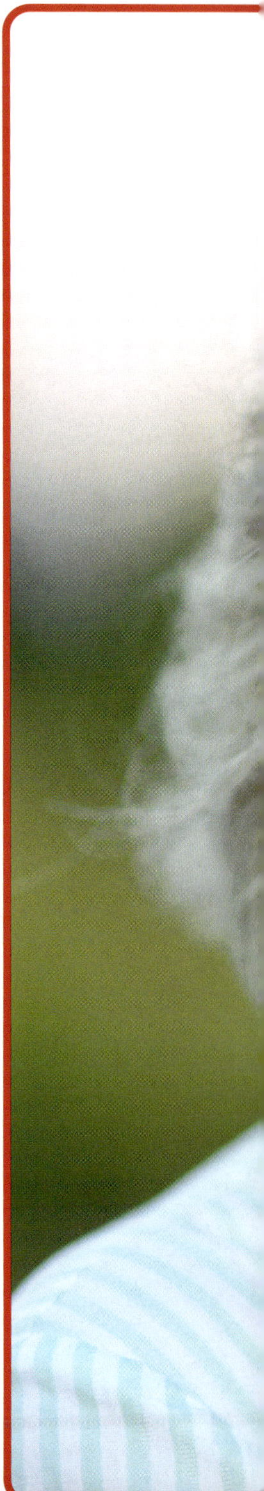

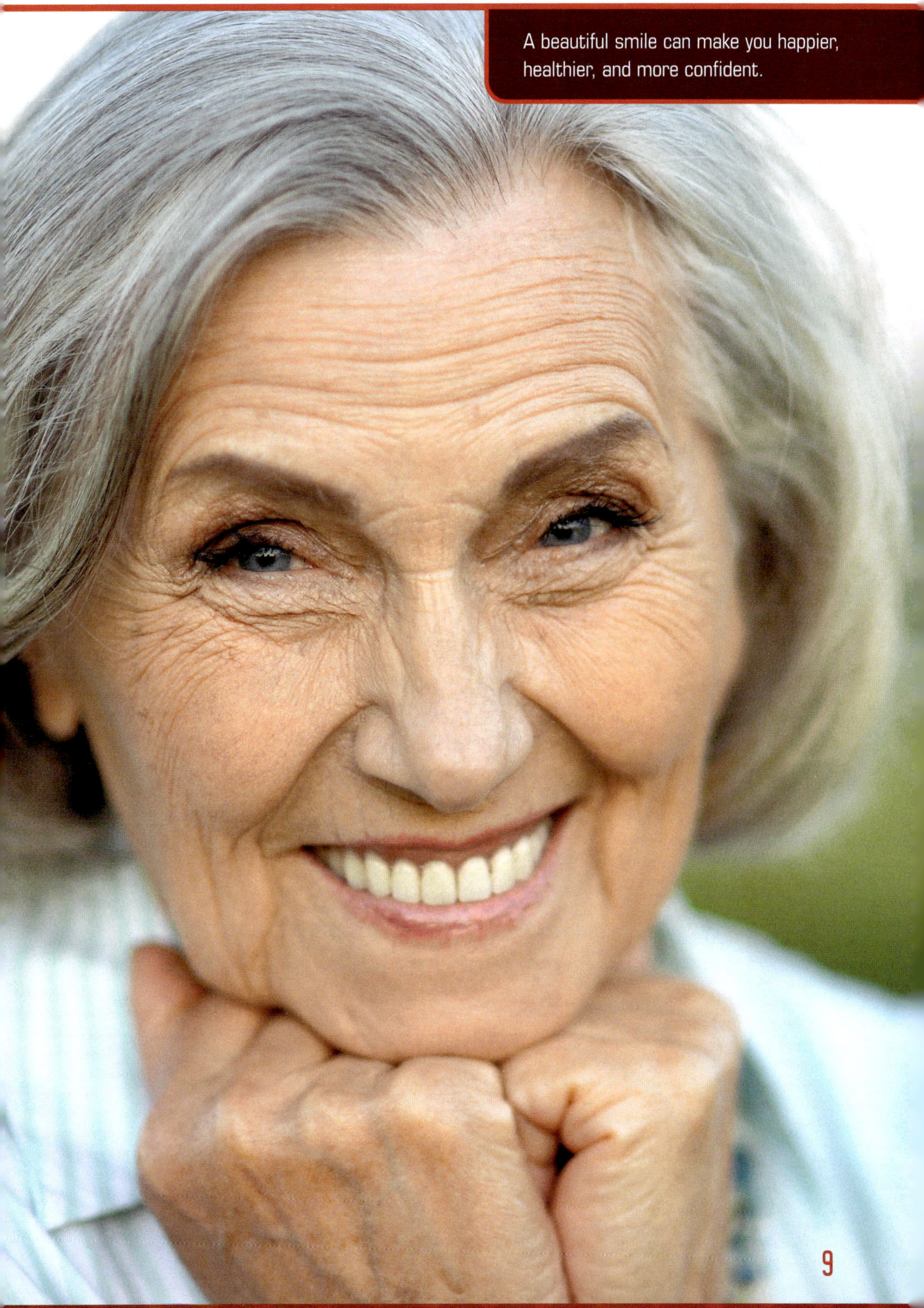

A beautiful smile can make you happier, healthier, and more confident.

CHAPTER ONE

WHAT DO THEY DO?

People might associate a dental hygienist with cleaning teeth. Of course, that's a big part of their job, but it's only the beginning. They're not just cleaning teeth to make them pretty—they're trained health care professionals doing an important job. In addition to cleaning and treating teeth, dental hygienists educate their patients about dental health and hygiene practices.

TREATING THE WHOLE PERSON

Although many people visit the dental clinic because they want their teeth to look nice, a healthy mouth is more than shiny teeth. A healthy mouth involves everything in and around the mouth: teeth, gums, tongue, jawbone, and all the tissue inside the mouth. A hygienist is concerned not only with dental (teeth) health, but also with oral (mouth) health.

Oral health affects a person's overall well-being because the parts of the body are connected. Bacteria that live in the mouth can get into the bloodstream. These bacteria may be harmless in the mouth but can cause problems in other places. And diseases in other parts of the body can show up in the mouth. For example, diabetes can cause dry mouth. Smoking can cause cancer in the mouth and throat. So dental hygienists examine their patients carefully.

They usually ask questions about patients' medical history. They find out if they're taking any medications. People with heart conditions sometimes take prescription blood thinners. This means they can bleed heavily from even a small cut. Dentists and hygienists need to be aware of things like that so they can plan treatment and take appropriate precautions. Sometimes they take the patient's temperature, blood pressure, and pulse. They simply want to make sure that whatever they do for the patient doesn't interfere with any condition the patient may have.

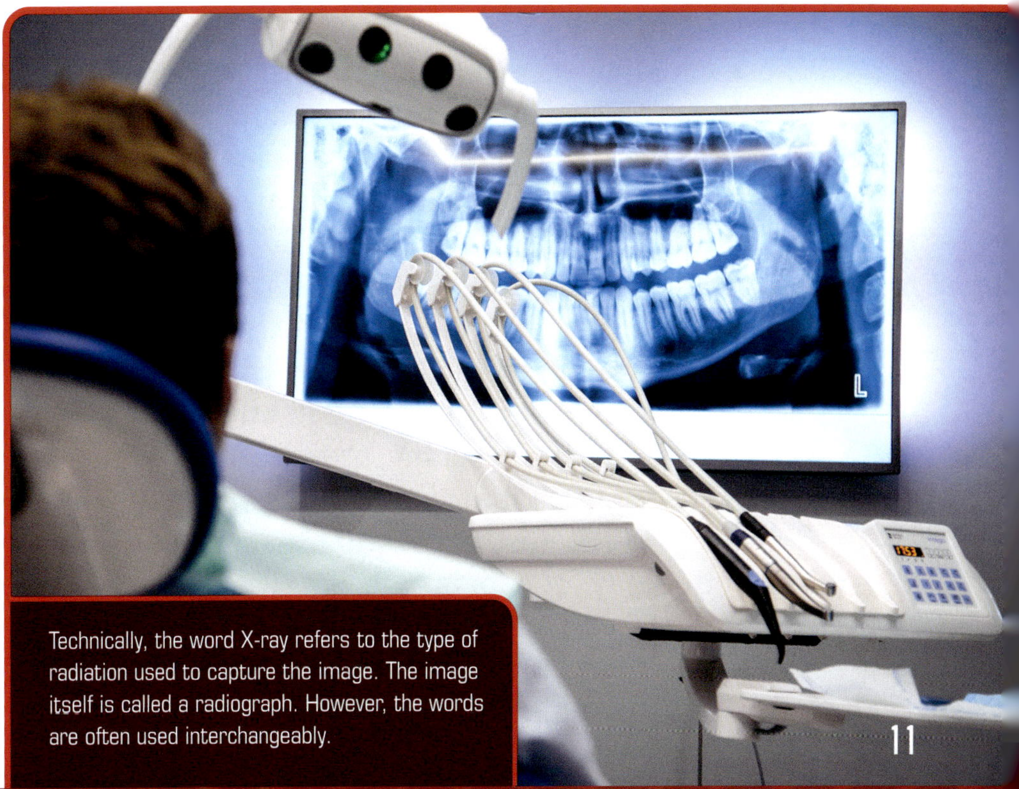

Technically, the word X-ray refers to the type of radiation used to capture the image. The image itself is called a radiograph. However, the words are often used interchangeably.

When hygienists examine their patients' mouths, they look for more than evidence of decay or other problems with their teeth. They see if the gums are healthy—pink and tight around the teeth—or red and puffy. They may wiggle the teeth to check how firm the gums are. They look carefully for sores, lumps, and anything abnormal. These could signal an infection. Feeling under a patient's chin tells the hygienist if lymph nodes are healthy. Swelling or tenderness in this area can be signs of throat or oral cancer. For more detailed examination, hygienists take X-rays, also called radiographs, of their patients' teeth.

AN OUNCE OF PREVENTION

Generally, you spend much more of your time in a dental clinic dealing with a hygienist than a dentist. After evaluating their patients' health, hygienists provide preventive dental care. Preventive care is treatment designed to help stop problems before they begin. Most tooth problems begin with cavities, and cavities begin with plaque.

Dental plaque is a soft, thin film that attaches itself to teeth. It is made up of microscopic bits of food, mucus, and dead cells from inside the mouth. Bacteria also live in plaque, feeding on sugars in food. The bacteria in plaque produce acids and toxins. The acids eat into enamel, the hard coating that covers the teeth. This is what makes cavities and tooth decay. The toxins attack the gums, and, over time, they can cause periodontal disease.

If the soft plaque stays on the teeth for more than a day, it combines with minerals in the mouth

to form tartar, also called calculus. Tartar often looks yellow or brown. It's hard and rough—just right for the sticky plaque with all its bacteria.

Plaque can be removed by proper brushing and flossing, but tartar can't. Tartar has to be scraped off. It must be removed carefully with special tools so that the scraping doesn't damage the teeth or injure the gums. Dental hygienists are trained to clean both plaque and tartar off teeth. In this way they help their patients prevent cavities, decay, and gum disease.

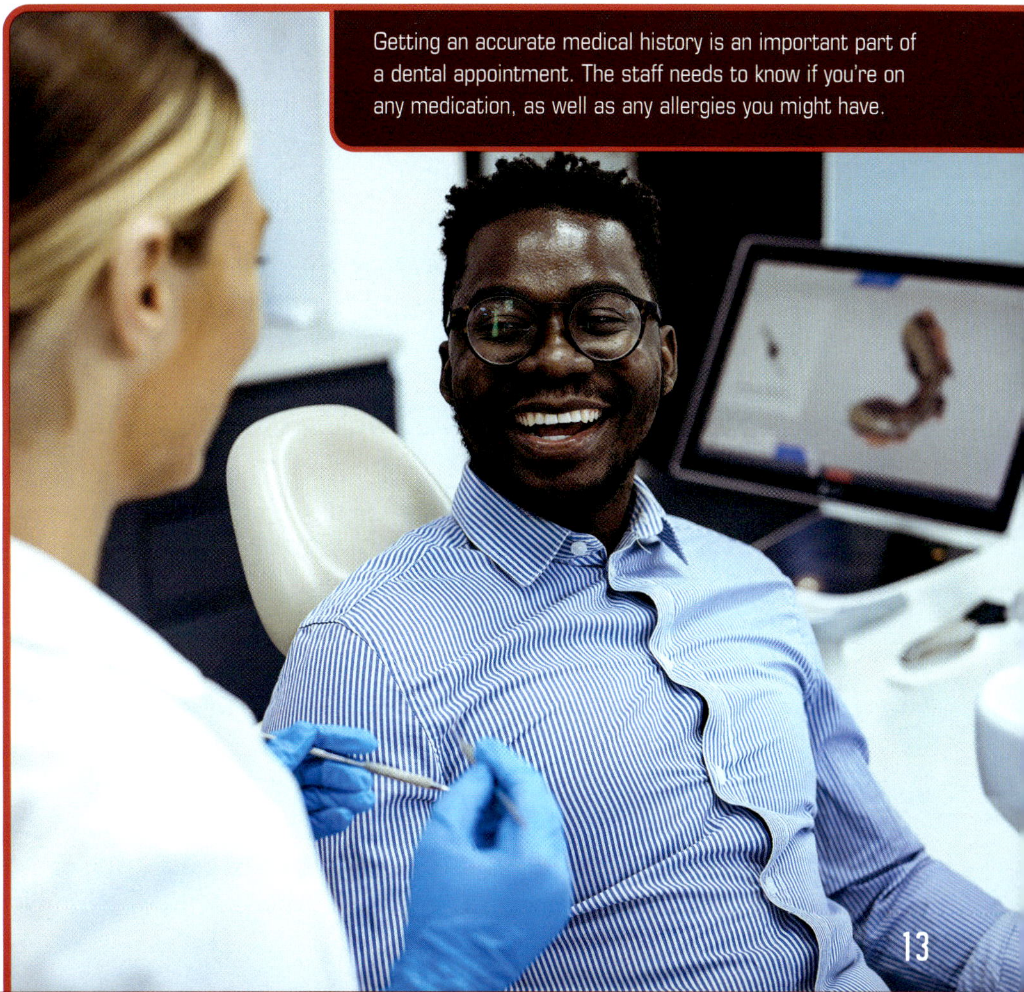

Getting an accurate medical history is an important part of a dental appointment. The staff needs to know if you're on any medication, as well as any allergies you might have.

Another way hygienists provide preventive dental care is by applying fluoride and sealants to children's teeth. Fluoride strengthens teeth, making decay less likely. Sealants are plastic coatings that fill the pits or grooves that are in some teeth. The pits are hard to clean with simple brushing, but the plastic seals them so no bacteria can get in. This is helpful, as kids tend to not be very careful about brushing their teeth. Baby teeth need to be taken care of so the gums are healthy when the permanent teeth grow in.

EDUCATION

A big part of a dental hygienist's job is teaching people to take good care of their own teeth. Generally, people visit the dental clinic once or twice a year. They need to take care of their teeth at home every single day. A hygienist can help people have healthy mouths by teaching them how to care for their own teeth and gums.

Hygienists show their patients the most effective ways to brush and floss. They explain the differences in toothbrushes, pastes, and gels and help their patients decide which products are best for them. They show their patients various tools for keeping their mouths healthy, and they demonstrate how to use them. Hygienists also explain how what people put in their mouths—food, cigarettes, chewing gum—affects their oral health. Chewing on things like pen caps or sucking your thumb can also affect your teeth. They encourage people to choose healthy foods and healthy habits. Some dental hygienists go to schools, libraries, and community events to promote good oral practices.

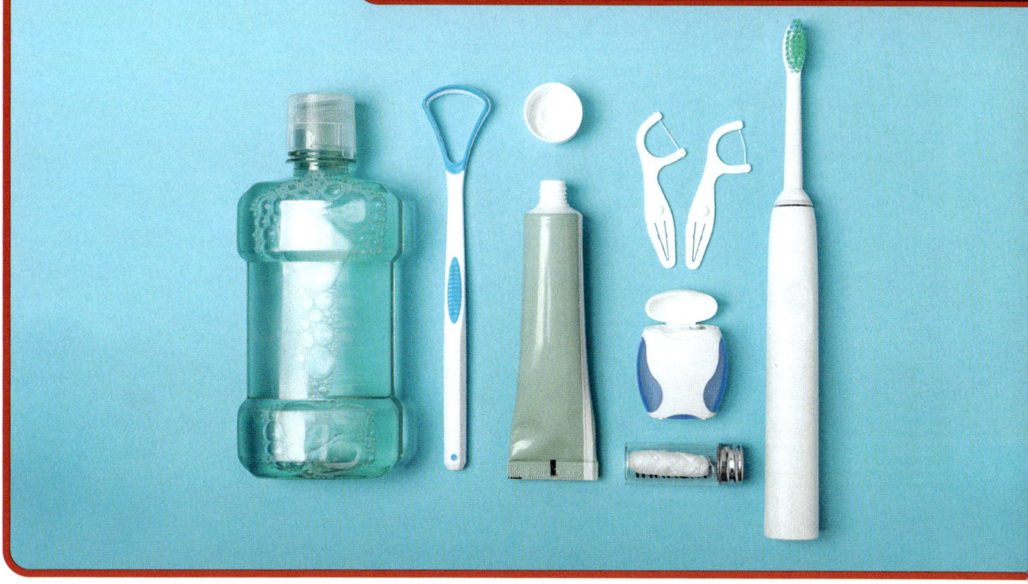

Dental hygienists teach people what sort of products they should use on their teeth and the best way to use them.

PREVENTATIVE DENTAL SERVICES

In general, hygienists provide preventive dental services and dentists provide therapeutic services. Therapeutic services are procedures aimed at healing. Hygienists try to prevent problems from happening in the first place. Dentists repair the ones that do occur despite everyone's best efforts. But in some cases, hygienists perform some simple therapeutic procedures.

Hygienists may do root planing and scaling. These are deep cleanings that remove plaque and tartar from the lower portions of the teeth, the parts below the gum line, around the tooth roots. They use local anesthetic is used for these procedures. It may take more than one appointment to treat all the patient's teeth. Scaling scrapes away bacteria

THE FATHER OF DENTAL HYGIENE

Although modern or medically based dentistry has been practiced since about the 16th century, up until the 20th century most people only saw a dentist when a tooth caused them pain. Most dentistry was based around the idea of removing the painful tooth and constructing false teeth.

In 1906, a Connecticut dentist, Dr. Alfred Fones, thought he knew why people's teeth went bad and why their gums hurt: they were covered with plaque and tartar. He tried to tell other dentists and doctors that if people cleaned their teeth, their mouths would feel better, and their teeth would last longer. Unfortunately, other doctors didn't see the value of preventive care.

So, Fones set out to prove his theory. He used some of the teeth he had pulled from his patients to make a model of a mouth. He put plaster of Paris around the base of the teeth to look and feel like tartar and stains. Then he taught his cousin, Irene Newman, how to clean the teeth.

Before long, other dentists saw that Fones's patients had healthier mouths than their patients. When Fones opened his first school of dental hygiene in 1913, dental professors from Harvard, Yale, and other well-known universities volunteered to teach. In the first year, 27 female students graduated. The Bridgeport School District hired most of them. They cleaned school children's teeth, which greatly reduced tooth decay and cavities. This helped lend credence to the new field of dental hygiene. In 1917, Newman became the first licensed dental hygienist in the world.

A common tool hygienists use is red tablets that show any plaque left on teeth after brushing. This helps people learn how to brush their teeth better.

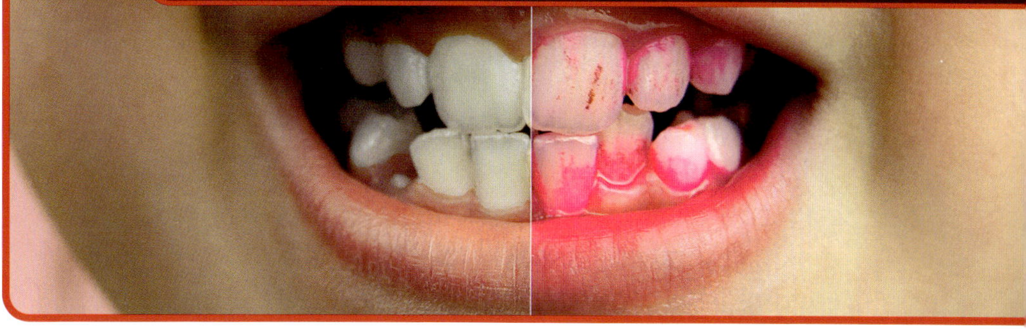

and toxins; root planing smooths the surface of the root so bacteria don't stick as well. People with gum problems often need to have such deep cleaning.

Each U.S. state has its own rules about what dental hygienists are allowed to do. In some states, they can mix the materials for fillings and put them in patients' teeth. In other states, they can put in temporary fillings, but only a dentist can insert permanent fillings. Some hygienists can give their patients anesthetics. Hygienists sometimes assist dentists when they perform oral surgery. Although they can't perform any part of the surgery, some hygienists can take out the stitches after the surgery is over. In some places, there is yet another type of dental professional called a dental therapist. They have more training than a hygienist—usually a master's degree—but less than a dentist.

WHAT ELSE?

After each appointment, hygienists need to clean and sanitize their workspace. In some practices, a dental assistant might do some of this work. Because so many germs are present inside peoples' mouths, even before the COVID-19 pandemic, hygienists were especially careful of sanitation. Hygienists also must carefully record each patient's condition and progress. Keeping patients' charts up to date is an important part of their job.

Then they must set up their space for the next appointment. They must sharpen and sterilize their instruments and make sure there's plenty of the correct PPE available for the next client. They must check the next patient's chart and make sure they have everything they need. For instance, if the next appointment is a child, they might select different educational materials than they would for an adult.

As you can see, a dental hygienist wears many hats—cleaner, dentist, technician, teacher, and record keeper.

SHAME FREE DENTISTRY

Going to the dentist isn't anyone's favorite thing to do. However, some people avoid it more than others. There are many reasons why someone might avoid visiting the dentist. These can include:

- cost/not having insurance
- fear of pain or having had painful procedures in the past
- embarrassment about the state of their teeth
- fear that the staff will lecture or berate them

Fortunately, modern dentistry tries to correct many of these issues so people can get the care they need. People without insurance can often find neighborhood health clinics where they can be seen by a dental hygienist or volunteer dentist.

People who are sensitive to pain or have had bad experiences can speak to someone before their treatment and make a plan. They might be prescribed medication to help them relax, and there are anesthetics available, so they won't feel pain. For people who are upset by the noise of dental equipment, noise-canceling headphones are available to help them relax.

Some people are embarrassed by the condition of their teeth. However, the staff is more interested in correcting their problems than commenting on them. After all, that's their job—to fix their clients' teeth.

Finally, most dental professionals now realize that lecturing their clients is a great way to lose them! They want you to visit them to get proper care for your teeth and mouth and will work to make sure you're comfortable, no matter what past experiences you might have had.

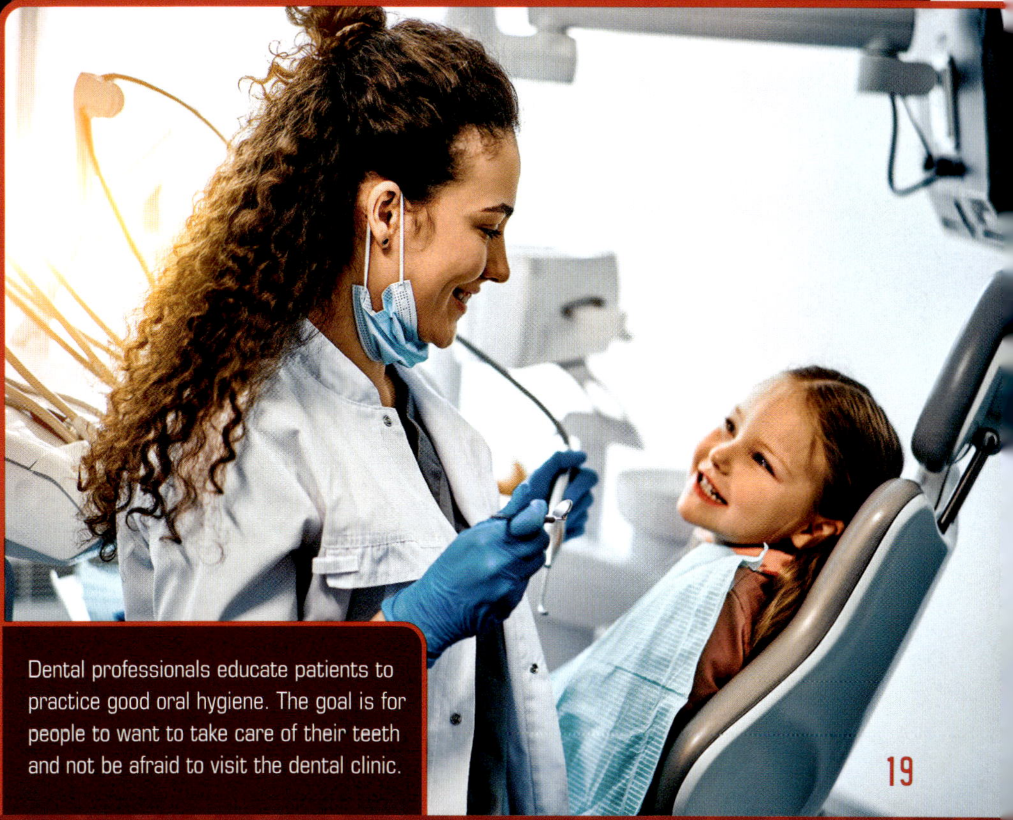

Dental professionals educate patients to practice good oral hygiene. The goal is for people to want to take care of their teeth and not be afraid to visit the dental clinic.

CHAPTER TWO

SO MANY OPTIONS!

A career as a dental hygienist can be much more than just cleaning teeth in a dental clinic. The American Dental Hygienists' Association (ADHA) lists seven career paths for dental hygienists: clinician, corporate, public health, researcher, educator, administrator, and entrepreneur. Although these paths involve different work settings and audiences, they all have the same goal: to help people have healthy mouths.

CLINICIAN

Every hygienist begins in the role of clinician. Clinicians work directly with patients. They're involved in helping people get well or stay well. Before hygienists can follow any other career path, they must thoroughly understand dental hygiene. They must practice evaluating patients, providing preventive care, teaching patients about oral health, and perhaps performing some basic therapeutic procedures.

Most hygienists remain in the career of clinician. They enjoy working directly with people. After all, most became hygienists because they wanted to help people. About 93 percent of all hygienists in the United States are clinicians in

Most hygienists will spend their entire career working directly with patients.

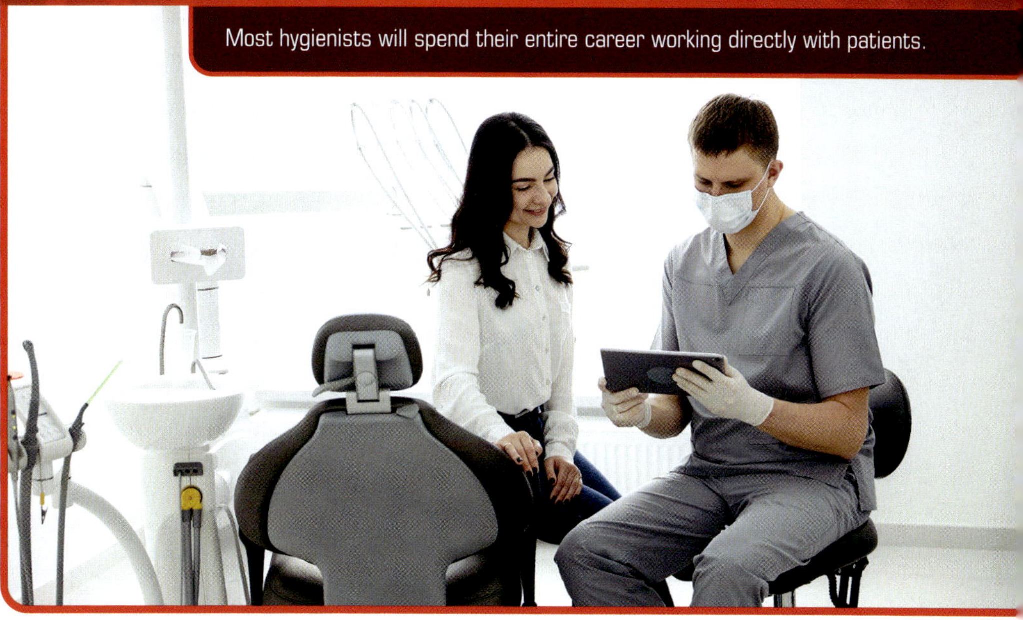

dental offices, according to the BLS. Another 1 percent work in doctors' offices. All these hygienists work in private practice, which means patients pay them either directly or through insurance. Other clinicians work in public health settings.

CORPORATE

Some dental hygienists leave clinical practice to work for oral health care companies. Several options are available to hygienists as managers and consultants in companies that make dental products. They might advise the people developing the products because they understand how the products will affect both clinicians and their patients. They could manage the public relations department because they are comfortable talking with dentists and hygienists. Some manage sales departments, helping salespeople learn how to present the products. They also make good salespeople for companies that make oral care products. Some of these career paths require additional schooling, either in advanced dental hygienics or in business—sometimes both.

PUBLIC HEALTH

Some hygienists work in community settings. Community settings are schools, clinics, prisons and juvenile halls, homes for the elderly and people with disabilities, military bases, and Indian reservations. Each of these is its own little community. In community settings, hygienists are paid not by their patients, but by government agencies or nonprofit groups. Patients in community settings often can't afford to pay for oral health care. In places with low incomes or high unemployment rates, people may not have insurance, and those who do may not have coverage that includes dental care. There may be local issues that affect their health, such as poor water supplies. Community-based dental service is called public health dentistry to distinguish it from private practice dentistry.

Hygienists in public dental health think of the community as their patient, rather than just the individuals in the community. So, in addition to the normal clinician duties, public health hygienists do outreach and dental health screenings. Outreach is going out into the community, talking to people about oral health and persuading them to come in to the clinic to receive care. Screening is examining people to see what their dental needs are. Many hygienists who work in community settings are especially happy they are able to teach and help people who would not have dental care without them. Often this work requires a more advanced education such as a bachelor's degree.

RESEARCHER

One other job option for educators and hygienists is research. Research generally takes place in a lab. Instead of working with a regular clientele of patients, researchers work with other researchers or perhaps small, carefully selected test groups. Dentists and people who make dental equipment and materials do research to make their practice and instruments better. Dental sealants, electric toothbrushes, and fluoride toothpaste are all the results of research. Two types of research for dental hygienists are clinical research and product development.

Another current research project is looking into whether wearing masks for extended periods of time during the pandemic trapped bacteria in people's mouths, leading to tooth decay.

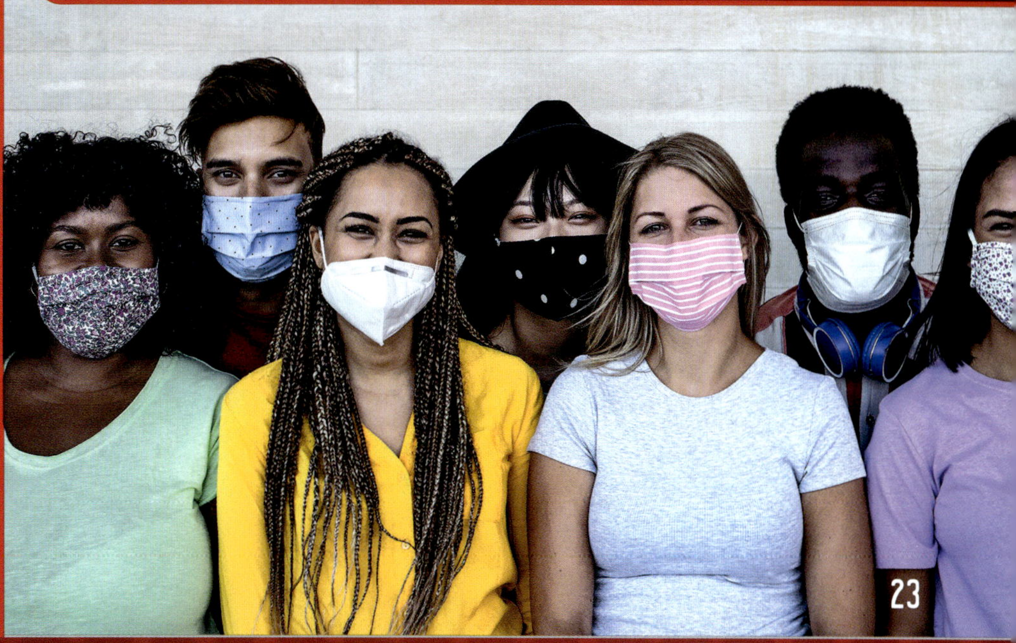

Clinical research has to do with everyday practices of oral health. Clinical researchers study the effects of food, medicines, and diseases on teeth and gums. For example, currently there is research about the effects of the virus that causes COVID-19 on people with poor oral health. They look for ways to improve the techniques clinicians use. They try to discover the early signs of oral cancer and gum disease. Other researchers design equipment, appliances, drugs, and other products that make it easier for dentists and hygienists to do their jobs and for ordinary people to take good care of their oral health.

Dental research takes teams of people. For example, consider a simple study on whether Toothbrush A cleans teeth better than Toothbrush B. Someone must design the study, and someone must find people to be in it—lots of people. Someone must distribute the toothbrushes and make sure everyone is using them the same way. Yet more people need to record the results, analyze them, and figure out what they mean. And this is a simple study!

Sometimes researchers must go back and take another look at past research projects. For example, at one point, companies that manufacture personal care items such as toothpaste and facial cleansers were adding microbeads to their products. The beads acted as a mild abrasive to help clean skin and teeth. However, new research suggests that plastic microbeads cause terrible environmental problems, and now they're banned. So now researchers must find something else that serves the same purpose but doesn't damage the environment.

Hygienists can find research opportunities at government agencies, health care companies, and businesses that manufacture health care products. Some universities have research departments. Hygienists working as clinicians or educators can also participate in research.

EDUCATOR

Teaching is another avenue open to dental hygienists. Requirements can vary greatly, with some positions requiring a master's or even a doctoral degree. One path is in public schools. Hygienists can teach children how to care for their teeth as early as preschool. In elementary school, they can also explain the connection between what people eat and their oral health. In the upper grades, dental hygiene is often a part of science or health class. Some high schools have vocational courses that prepare students for jobs. Others have programs that introduce students to different careers. Any of these is a great opportunity for a hygienist educator.

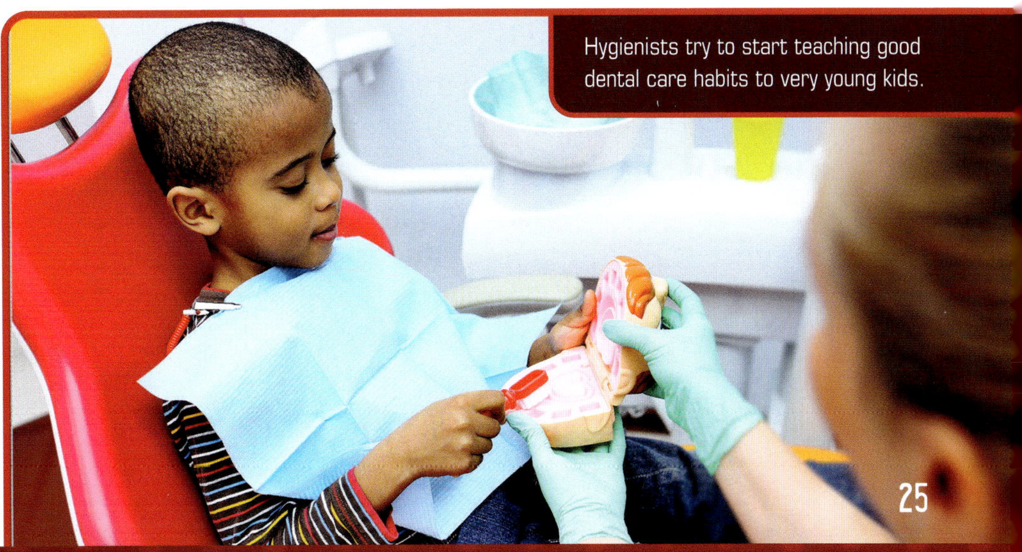

Hygienists try to start teaching good dental care habits to very young kids.

There will always be a need for experienced hygienists to train the next generation. Community colleges, technical colleges, dental schools, and four-year colleges have programs that prepare people to become dental hygienists. Most also have continuing education classes that are required for hygienists to stay up on the latest techniques.

Community settings have many needs for dental educators. Clinics often hire hygienists to conduct classes or seminars on dental health. Clinics and community organizations frequently have hygienists speak or demonstrate good oral care at health fairs and other neighborhood events.

Dental education is not all lecture and classroom instruction. Sometimes it is using a puppet, or singing songs, or even dressing up as "Myrtle the Molar." Many hygienists who choose education as a career path teach only part-time; the rest of the time they work as clinicians or in other jobs in the field. This is a good path for someone who wants more variety in their work life.

ADMINISTRATOR

Administrative positions require not just dental hygiene credentials, but also advanced business skills. Typically, these positions require a masters or doctoral degree. If a dental hygienist has skills in administration—in running things—they can manage a dental office. As managers, they take charge of scheduling, hiring, and day-to-day operations. Hygienists might also work as directors of community programs, research centers, or corporate sales directors for companies that sell oral care products.

ENTREPRENEUR

Hygienists with a good head for business might decide to start their own company or nonprofit organization. They might choose to open their own practice, rather than work in someone else's office. Or they might run a placement service, helping other hygienists find jobs.

TONYA RAY, CLINICIAN, EDUCATOR, AND MANAGER

All dental hygienists start out as clinicians, and some hold that position for their entire career. Others, such as Tonya Ray, are more adventurous.

Ray has traveled three different paths in her career as a dental hygienist. She began as a clinician in a school for people with developmental disabilities. She really enjoyed knowing she was helping her patients. Then she went back to school and became a teacher. She loved helping others become dental hygienists. While she was teaching, she also managed the school's dental clinic. After that, she became a manager for large companies that made dental products. She travels all over the country, using her skills as a hygienist as she meets people, trains them, and helps their businesses grow. Every job has brought new challenges and new rewards. And she has loved every one of them.

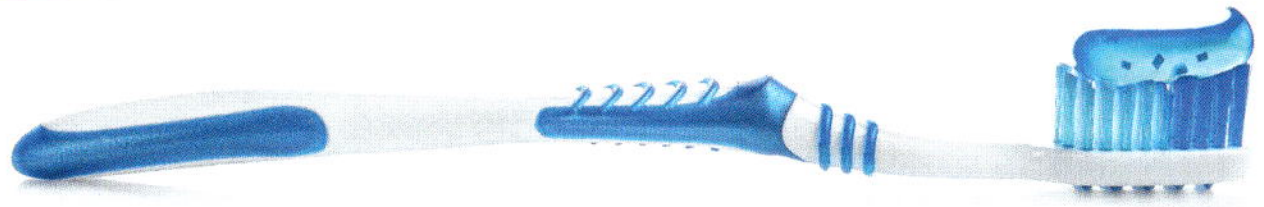

The best dental product doesn't do any good unless people buy it and use it. Dental hygienists help market new products to both industry professionals and the public.

A FLEXIBLE CAREER

The field of dental hygiene has many different job options, making it a good choice for a long-term career. Although all hygienists start out as clinicians, they have plenty of other options available. Hygienists can work full-time or part-time. They can work days or nights, weekdays or weekends. They can acquire further education and move on to become a teacher or researcher. Or they can divide their time and do more than one type of work. They can work in a small office with one dentist or in a large medical complex. They can specialize, caring for children, working for periodontists (those who treat gum conditions), or helping with oral surgery. They can choose private practice or public dental health.

Whatever career path they choose, most hygienists naturally become advocates for good oral health. They know the importance of oral health and they know how to achieve it. So, they automatically encourage others to brush and floss properly, visit their dentist regularly, and follow a healthy diet. Some go on to become professional advocates, working mainly in public health as patient advocates. Advocates help people recognize their health needs and work with them to meet those needs. They give them the education and connect them with the resources that will enable them to practice good oral health care. In some communities, patients have difficulty knowing how and where to get what they need. Advocates help them understand and access all that is available. Dental health care advocacy is very rewarding for hygienists who like helping people.

FORENSICS

One career path you might not automatically associate with dental hygienists is that of forensics. Forensic dentistry uses knowledge of teeth as legal evidence. Forensic dentistry teams often use dental information to identify a body. A forensic dentist can tell a lot about people by examining their teeth: how old they are, whether they are male or female, and what their race is. Sometimes they can tell if they were wealthy or poor, if they smoked, or if they took certain medicines or had certain diseases. Usually, they identify people by comparing their dental records with the physical evidence they find. Forensic dental teams have been invaluable in identifying victims of natural disasters such as hurricanes and tsunamis and identifying crime victims.

Hygienists make good members of forensic teams. They're used to spotting unusual traits in people's teeth. They're skilled in taking and understanding radiographs. They're accustomed to noticing and recording the tiniest details about their patients' teeth.

More than 140 forensic dentists worked on identifying bodies of victims following the September 11, 2001, terrorist attacks. Many hygienists who serve on forensic teams also work as clinicians, teachers, managers, or consultants.

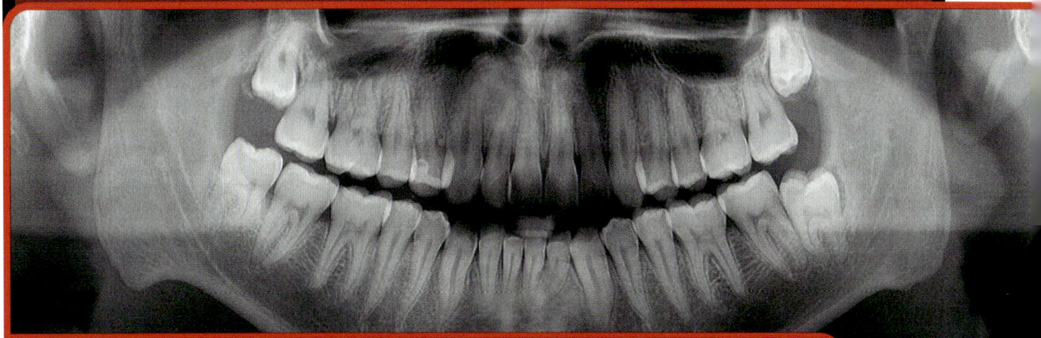

Forensic dentists provide invaluable aid to both criminal cases and disaster recovery.

CHAPTER THREE

TOOLS OF THE TRADE

Just as all dental hygienists start out as clinicians, they also all need to master the same basic tools. Some are hand tools that haven't changed much over time. Others are new digital technology. And others were invented by hygienists to help them do their job better.

Some tools are for diagnosing, or evaluating, patients' conditions; some are for cleaning teeth; and some are for keeping patients' mouths healthy.

PROBES

Some of the most familiar tools a dental hygienist uses in an exam are hand tools. One of these is called a dental probe, or explorer. As the name suggests, its purpose is to probe, or explore, the teeth and gums to see what condition they are in. Probes are thin, straight instruments with sharp, hooked ends. Some probes have hooks on only one end, and some have two curved ends, one slightly larger than the other. The curve lets the hygienist slip the probe around and between teeth. The hygienist pokes the teeth with the sharp end to find any decay. Tooth decay begins as soft spots on the tooth's enamel, and the spots are too tiny to see in the beginning. However, a trained hygienist can feel them with the probe.

Hygienists need good manual dexterity. They need to be able to feel tiny imperfections in teeth through the probes they're using. They also need to be very gentle when exploring teeth. If they're too rough, the sharp probe can turn a minor problem into a major one. Sometimes they can remove a slight bit of decay and repair the tooth with a fluoride treatment, but harsh probing can widen a small hole in the enamel.

The pointed end of the probe is also a measuring device. The hygienist uses it to measure the gum pocket—how far below the gum line the gum is separated from the teeth. This measurement tells how healthy the gums are.

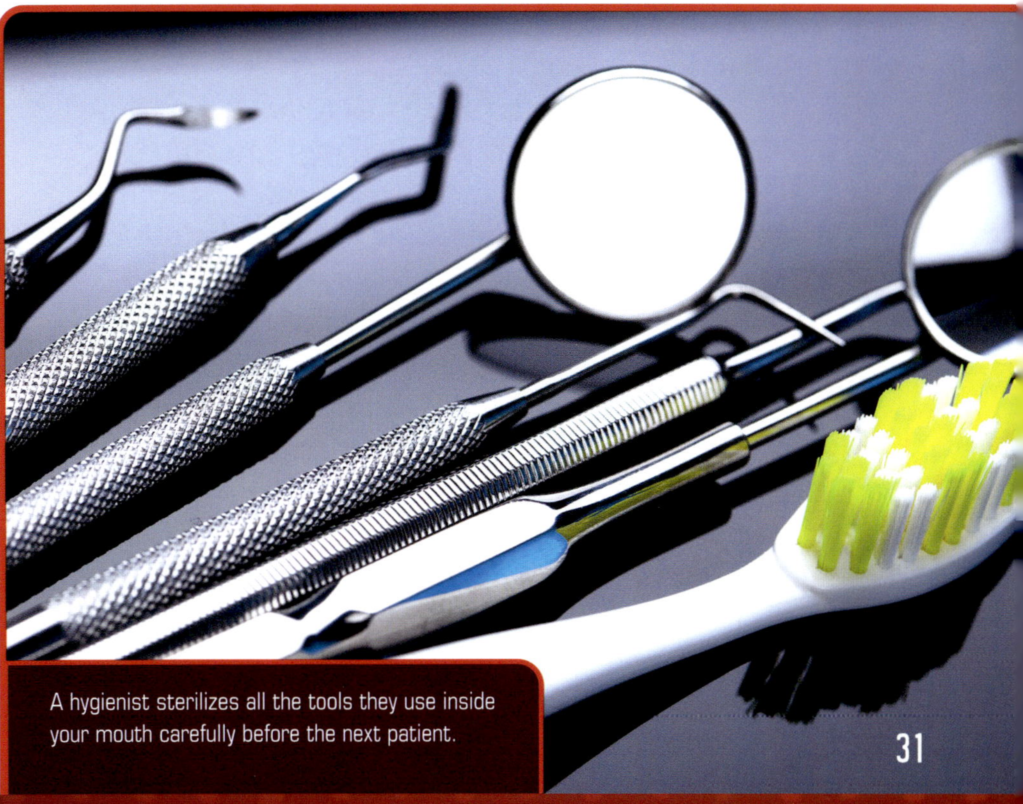

A hygienist sterilizes all the tools they use inside your mouth carefully before the next patient.

IMAGING

The best dental hygienist exploring with the finest dental probe can miss some problems. Some cavities are just too small to detect or located in places too difficult to reach. The hygienist can't see what is happening inside the gums. To discover what they can't see or feel with their instruments, hygienists take images of their patients' mouths.

These images are called X-rays or radiographs. technically, "X-ray" refers to the type of radiation that used to be used to obtain the image. The image itself is called a radiograph, or sometimes just a rad. X-rays are pictures of the insides of solid objects. Hygienists use them to spot any problems with their patients' teeth, gums, mouth, and jaw. They can show cavities, bone loss or damage, gum infections, and the positions of teeth that have not yet broken through the gums.

Traditional X-rays used to require film that took time to develop and resulted in printed images that had to be stored in file cabinets. If another doctor needed to see those images, they had to be packed up and shipped to another office. This took time and cost money. People were also concerned about the amount of radiation used in dental X-rays.

Today, many dental offices use a newer technology called digital radiography. Digital radiographs are taken, stored, and viewed with computers instead of film. The images can be seen and studied as soon as they're taken. If another doctor needs to consult on the case, the images can be sent over the internet in minutes. Some hygienists prefer digital radiography because it uses less radiation.

Hygienists not only take and process radiographs of their patients; they also interpret them. Radiographs are basically images of light and dark. Hygienists look at the pictures and figure out what they mean. For example, a dark spot on a white background may indicate a cavity on a tooth. Hygienists might notice problems, but they aren't licensed to diagnose them. When they identify a cavity or other issues, they point out their findings to a dentist and the dentist can treat the patient.

Digital X-ray images are ready to view right away and use considerably less radiation than traditional X-ray imaging.

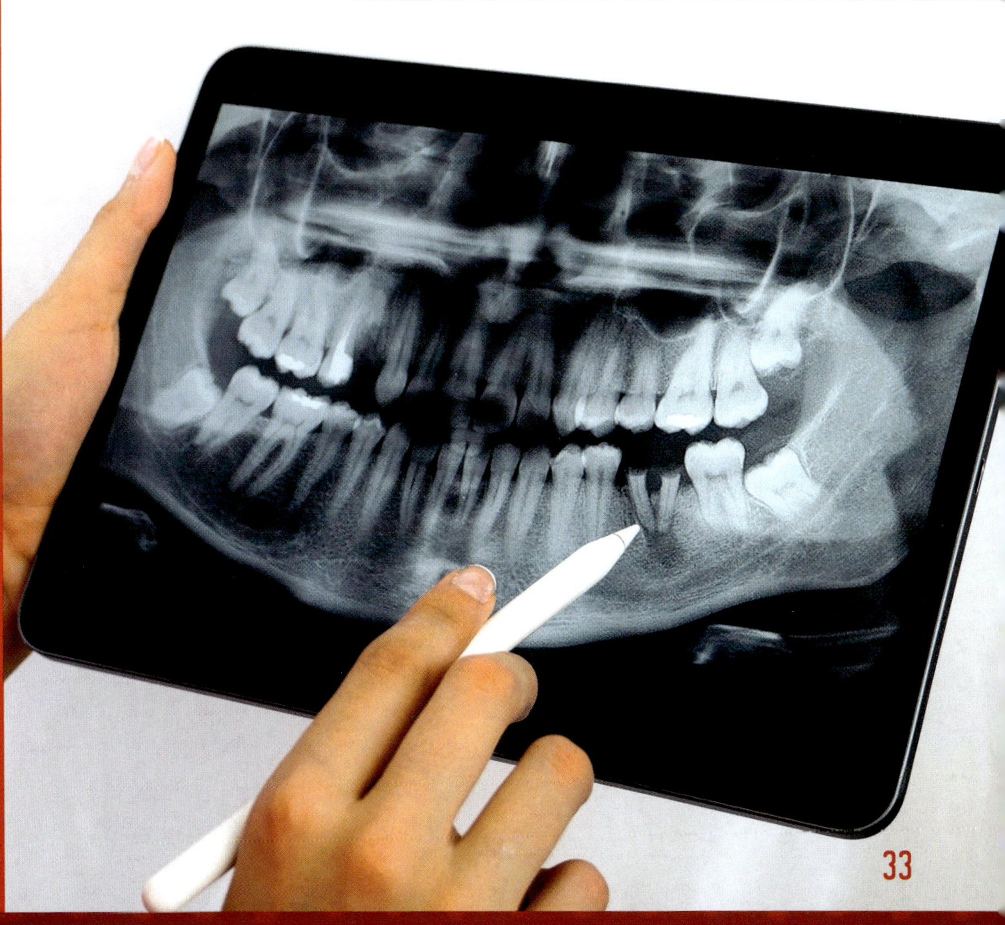

WHAT HAPPENS WHEN THE RIGHT TOOL DOESN'T EXIST?

Sometimes, the perfect tool for a job doesn't exist. Yet. Dental hygienists need to record information about their patients' teeth. They need to write down what they see in their patients' mouths, but they also need to keep their hands clean. If they use a pen or a computer to record the information and then go back to working on the patient, germs on the equipment could be transferred to the patient—or germs from the patient's mouth could be transferred to the office environment. Having an assistant transcribe the information meant having two people working on one patient at the same time.

Dental hygienist Becky Logue solved the problem. She invented the Dental R.A.T. (Remote Access Terminal). The R.A.T. is a large computer mouse placed on the floor and operated with the foot. It allows hygienists to put information into their computers without stopping their dental work and contaminating their hands. Logue got the idea when she saw her children play a game on a dance pad. Today, hundreds of hygienists use her invention.

Dentists recommend that patients have radiographs taken regularly, at least every few years, depending on the patient's age and the condition of their oral health. Patients undergoing orthodontic (tooth straightening) procedures might have images taken more often to see how their treatment is progressing. The images taken at different times can reveal conditions that may need attention. Hygienists are often responsible for keeping records of their patients' radiographs and knowing when to take new ones. Like most forms of records these days, digital X-rays are stored on a computer. The records as well as the images themselves are important in the evaluation aspect of the dental hygienist's job.

SCALERS

After the initial evaluation, the hygienist cleans the patient's teeth, removing the soft and hard deposits that build up on teeth. Cleaning tools are called scalers. Scalers look very much like probes, but their tips are very narrow triangular blades, rather than pointed ends. Hygienists use scalers to scrape plaque and tartar from teeth. They use different scalers—with their blades curved at various angles—so that they can reach around and between all the teeth. When they clean below the gum line, they switch to curettes. A curette is a scaler with a rounded tip that is gentle against the gum. These are all hand scalers.

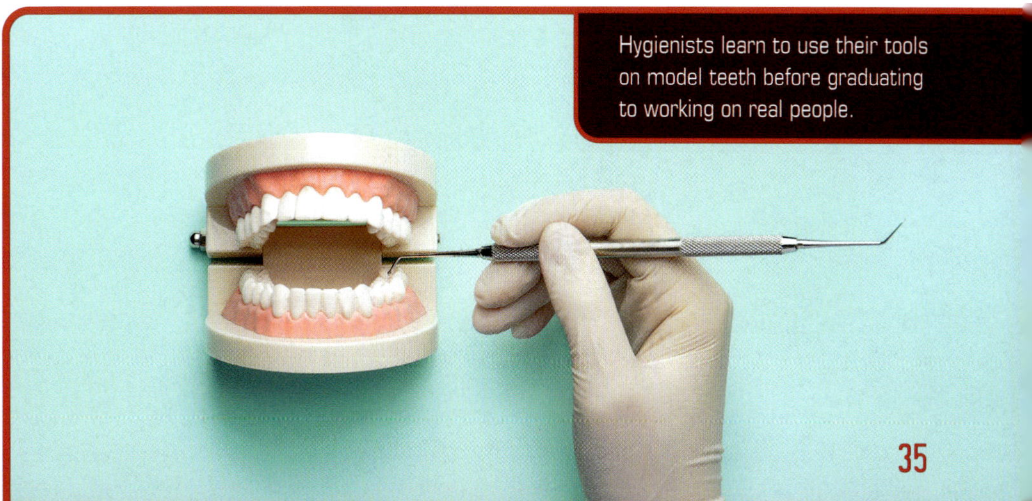

Hygienists learn to use their tools on model teeth before graduating to working on real people.

Hygienists may also use ultrasonic scalers. An ultrasonic scaler is a scaler that vibrates. Using an ultrasonic scaler is a little like using an electric toothbrush. The vibrations loosen built-up deposits faster than hand scaling. The hygienist removes the deposits by rinsing the teeth. Although they are faster and more comfortable for both patient and hygienist, ultrasonic scalers do not usually remove all tartar. Hygienists finish the cleaning with a hand scaler. These professional tools remove plaque and tartar that your toothbrush can't.

CLEANING AIDS

Probes and scalers are the primary instruments hygienists use, but other tools are also helpful. Probably the most familiar is the small mouth mirror on a long handle. The mirror is set on an angle to help the hygienist see behind teeth. They enable the

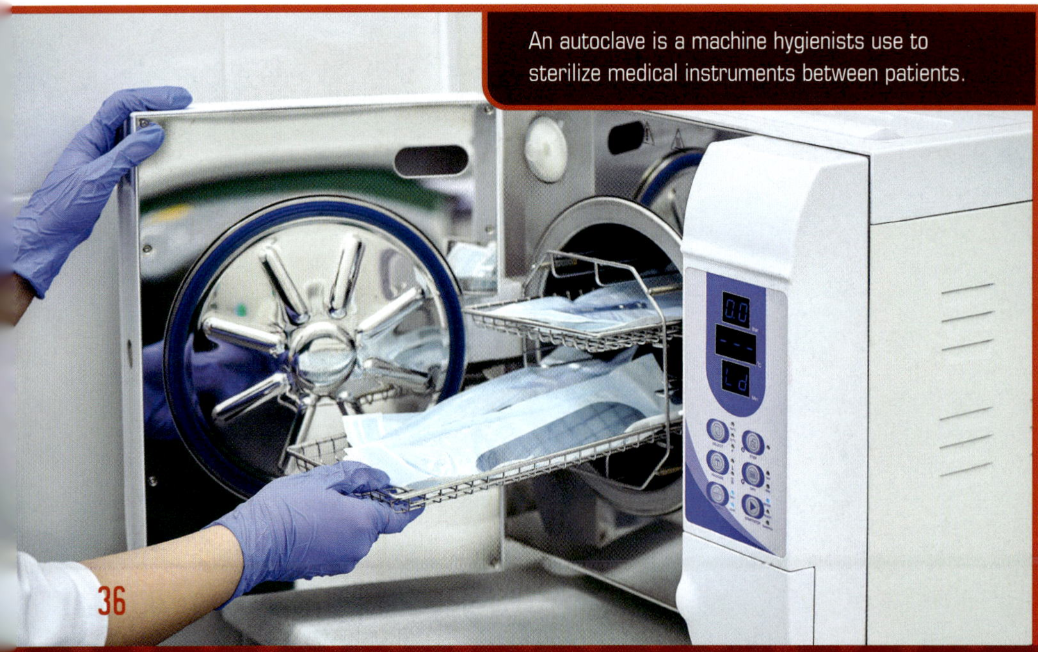

An autoclave is a machine hygienists use to sterilize medical instruments between patients.

hygienist to see all the surfaces of any tooth and reflect light where it's needed. Hygienists also use mirrors to hold the patient's tongue or lip out of their way so they can see the teeth better.

As hygienists scrape plaque and tartar from their patients' teeth, they use a water/air syringe to remove the debris. The syringe shoots a blast of air, a stream of water, or both. The air and/or water flush the unwanted material away from the clean tooth.

But the debris must go somewhere. So, the hygienist uses a dental vacuum to suction it out of patients' mouths. The vacuum also removes blood and excess saliva. Sometimes a curved hose is attached to the vacuum and hooked loosely over the patient's lower lip. This allows hygienists to keep working on patients without having to stop frequently to suction their mouths.

After cleaning the teeth, the hygienist polishes them. The polish is applied with an electric instrument that rotates against the teeth. The purpose of polishing is not to make the teeth shine; it is to make them smooth so that it is more difficult for plaque to stick to them. It also removes any remaining specks of plaque.

Keeping patients healthy requires that hygienists do their jobs in a super-clean environment. That means they must sanitize their rooms between patients. They spray chairs, lights, trays, countertops, and hoses with disinfectant. They wipe everything down and clean all their equipment. To make sure no bacteria remain, they sterilize their instruments in an autoclave. An autoclave uses steam under pressure to kill any contaminants. In some practices, a dental assistant might do some of this work.

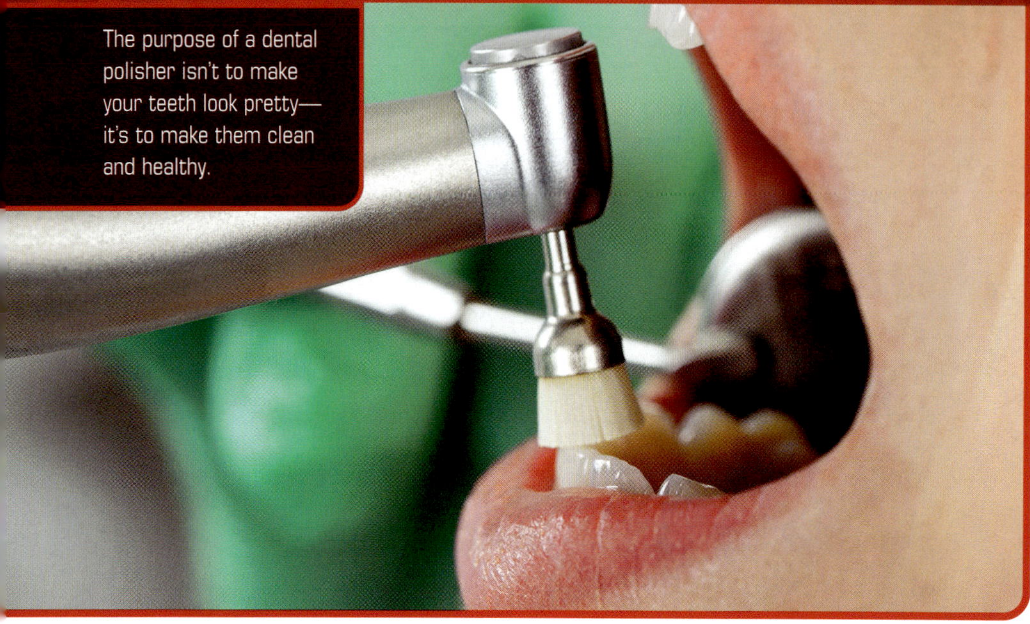

The purpose of a dental polisher isn't to make your teeth look pretty—it's to make them clean and healthy.

WORK SKILLS AND PEOPLE SKILLS

A dental hygienist training program teaches technical skills, but a successful candidate needs to possess certain qualities. They need to have good finger dexterity. That is, they must be able to hold small instruments in the fingers of one hand and move them carefully, gently, and firmly in tight spaces. They also need very good near vision and they need to combine finger dexterity with good vision: the job demands excellent eye-hand coordination.

In addition to physical abilities, hygienists need people skills. Some people are nervous when they come to a dentist's office, and a hygienist is often the first clinician they see. The hygienist needs to put patients at ease and make them feel comfortable. They need to listen to patients so they can understand their needs. They need to be able to explain the procedures they plan to do clearly and answer any questions the patient has.

Hygienists must be detail oriented. That means they pay attention to small items. They not only have to notice tiny problems in their patients' mouths and slight differences on radiographs, but they also must record much of what they see and do.

They need to be organized. Patient records need to be kept up to date and orderly, so other members of the team can find information when they need it. They must keep track of their tools and all the supplies they use.

What's more, being a dental hygienist requires a great deal of knowledge and technical skills. These are gained through professional training.

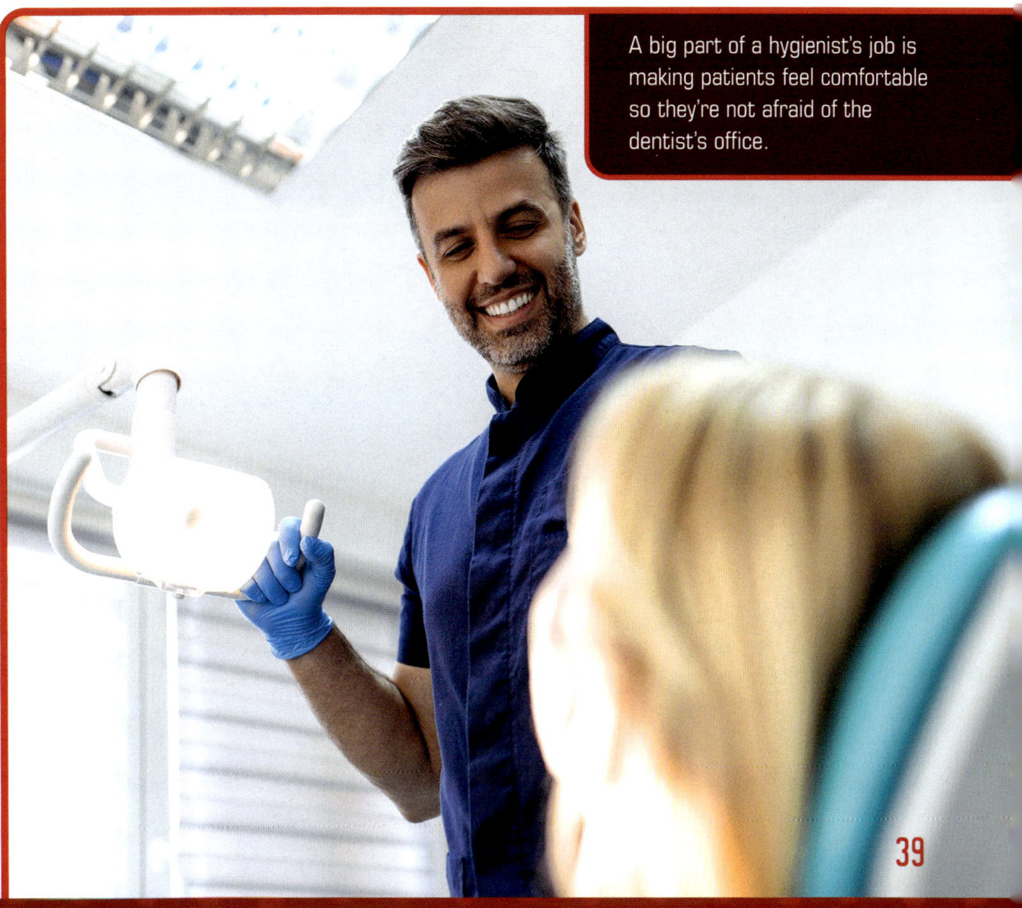

A big part of a hygienist's job is making patients feel comfortable so they're not afraid of the dentist's office.

A BRIEF HISTORY OF DENTISTRY

Did you know that one of the earliest references to dentistry dates all the way back to 5,000 BCE? An ancient Sumerian text lists "tooth worms" as the cause of tooth decay. This idea was accepted for centuries. Ancient Egyptians, Greeks, and Romans wrote about treating teeth and jaw fractures. A Chinese text from about the year 700 CE describes the use of silver paste for fillings.

From the 13th through the 16th centuries in Europe, barbers practiced dentistry. It mostly consisted of pulling painful teeth. During the 18th century, people began to consider dentistry a medical practice. Scientists developed crowns and dentures The first dental chair was built in 1790 and the first reclining dental chair in 1832.

Drs. Chapin A. Harris and Horace H. Hayden founded the Baltimore College of Dental Surgery, the world's first dental college, in 1840. This was also when the Doctor of Dental Surgery (DDS) degree was established. The American Dental Association (ADA) began operating in 1859.

In 1869, Dr. Robert Tanner Freedman became the first Black American to earn a dental degree. He graduated from Harvard University Dental School. The first Black American woman to graduate from dental school was Dr. Ida Gray in 1890.

German chemist Alfred Einhorn invented Novocain in 1905. The Army Dental Corps formed in 1911, and the Naval Dental Corps in 1912. The first nylon toothbrush was marketed in 1938. Government officials first added fluoride to public water systems in 1945 and fluoride toothpaste became available for sale in 1950. The first commercial electric toothbrush debuted in 1960.

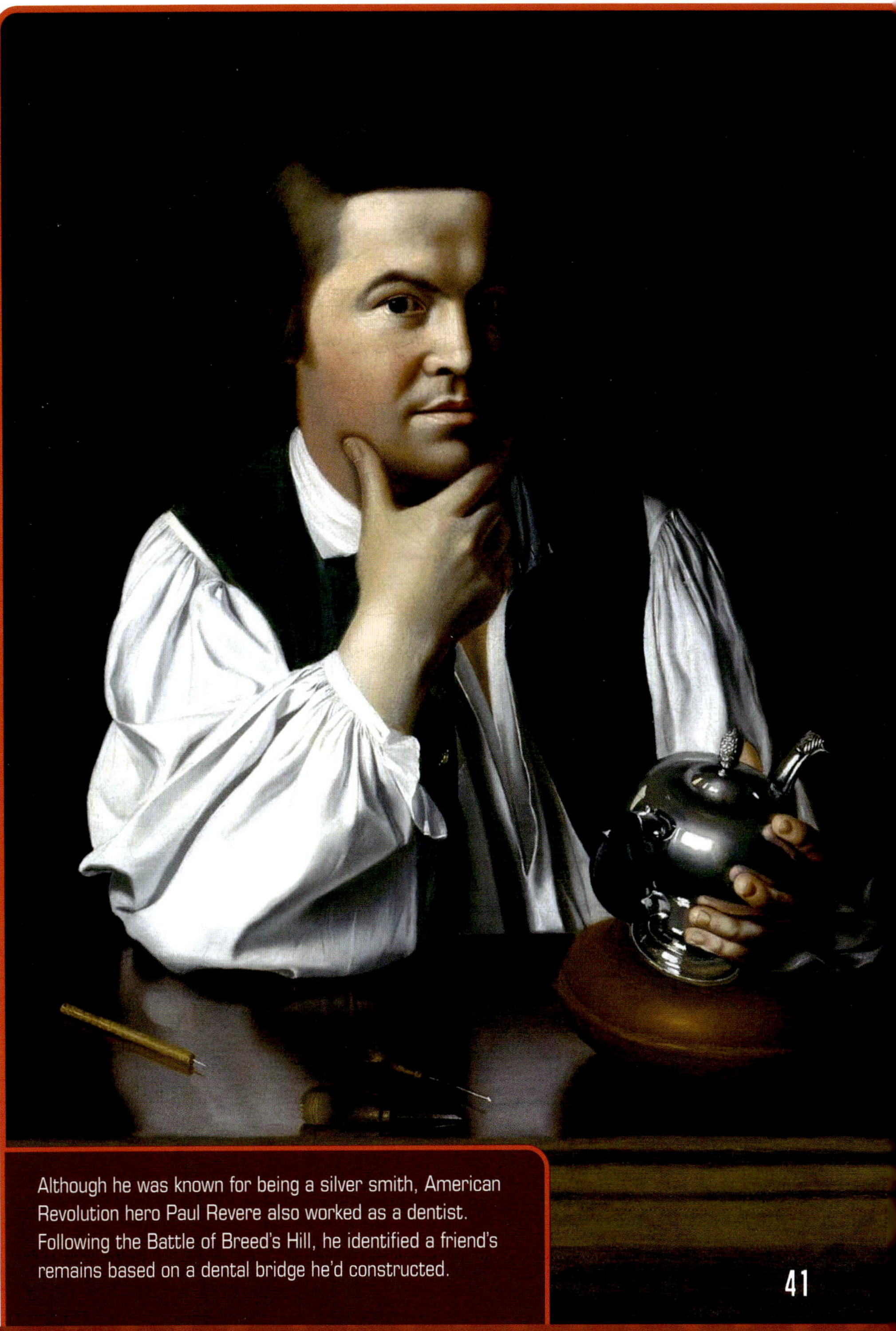

Although he was known for being a silver smith, American Revolution hero Paul Revere also worked as a dentist. Following the Battle of Breed's Hill, he identified a friend's remains based on a dental bridge he'd constructed.

CHAPTER FOUR

TRAINING AND EDUCATION

For many years, dental hygienists were considered "less" than dentists, especially since the vast majority are women. However, hygienists are skilled professionals that require at least one college degree and a license to practice. Dental hygienists must understand the structures of the mouth and jaw. They must know the relationship between oral health and the rest of the body. They need to know how diet and behavior affect teeth. They must learn how to use all the tools of the trade. They also must keep up with all the latest technological and clinical innovations. Dental hygiene is a profession that requires education, practice, and a state license.

The first requirement is education. The ADHA recognizes several types of training: entry-level, master's degree, degree completion, and online programs. In each type of program, students learn information and gain skills that enable them to qualify for different levels of dental hygienist jobs.

ENTRY-LEVEL TRAINING

The first step toward a career in dental hygiene is to take and pass the Admission Test for Dental

Hygiene. This is a standardized test administered by the ADA's Department of Testing Services. This helps schools make admissions decisions.

Entry-level programs are exactly what the name suggests: they give students enough training to enter the profession. Every hygienist enters the profession as a clinician. To get a job as a dental hygienist, a person must graduate from a dental education program that is accredited, or approved, by the ADA. The ADA sets the standards for hygienist education for the entire nation. Entry-level programs grant three types of proof that a graduate is ready to practice dental hygiene: a certificate, an associate's degree, and a bachelor's degree.

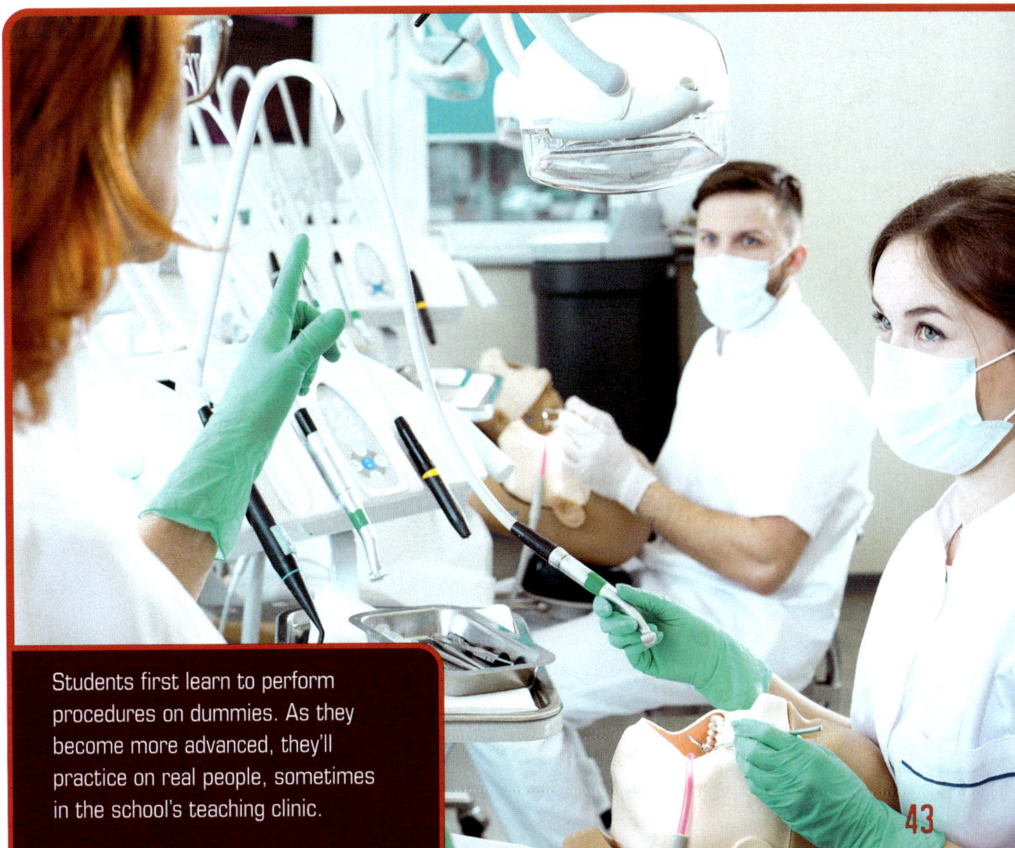

Students first learn to perform procedures on dummies. As they become more advanced, they'll practice on real people, sometimes in the school's teaching clinic.

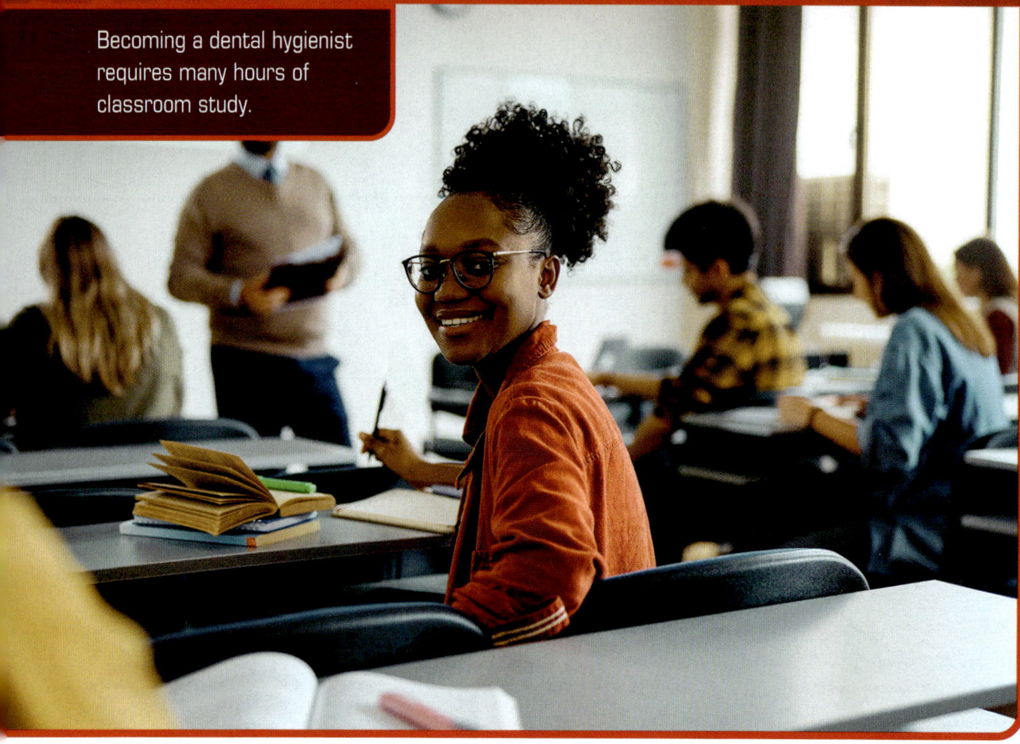

Becoming a dental hygienist requires many hours of classroom study.

The ADA has approved more than 300 entry-level training programs in the United States. In the vast majority, students earn an associate's degree—an Associate of Arts (AA), Associate of Science (AS), or Associate of Applied Science (AAS). They are offered at community colleges, also called junior colleges; technical colleges; and dental schools. In a few programs, students earn a certificate instead of a degree. Both the ADHA and ADA Commission on Dental Accreditation (CODA) websites have searchable databases to help students locate the best program for them.

Admission to some programs requires that the student has passed certain high school math and science classes and holds a valid CPR certification. Associate's degree and certificate programs basically require two years of study. The student spends about

2,300 hours in the classroom and about 500 hours in hands-on practice. The classroom time includes general courses that all college students take, such as English, math, and sociology. It also includes science classes; hygienists must know chemistry, anatomy, microbiology, physiology, and nutrition. A person working in other people's mouths must also know quite a bit about dental science. So, students in dental hygiene programs study the anatomy of the mouth and jaw and of the head and neck. They learn about teeth, gums, and diseases of the mouth. They learn how to manage pain, use different instruments, and take radiographs. Depending on the program, students may be required to pass each class with a certain grade to proceed in the program.

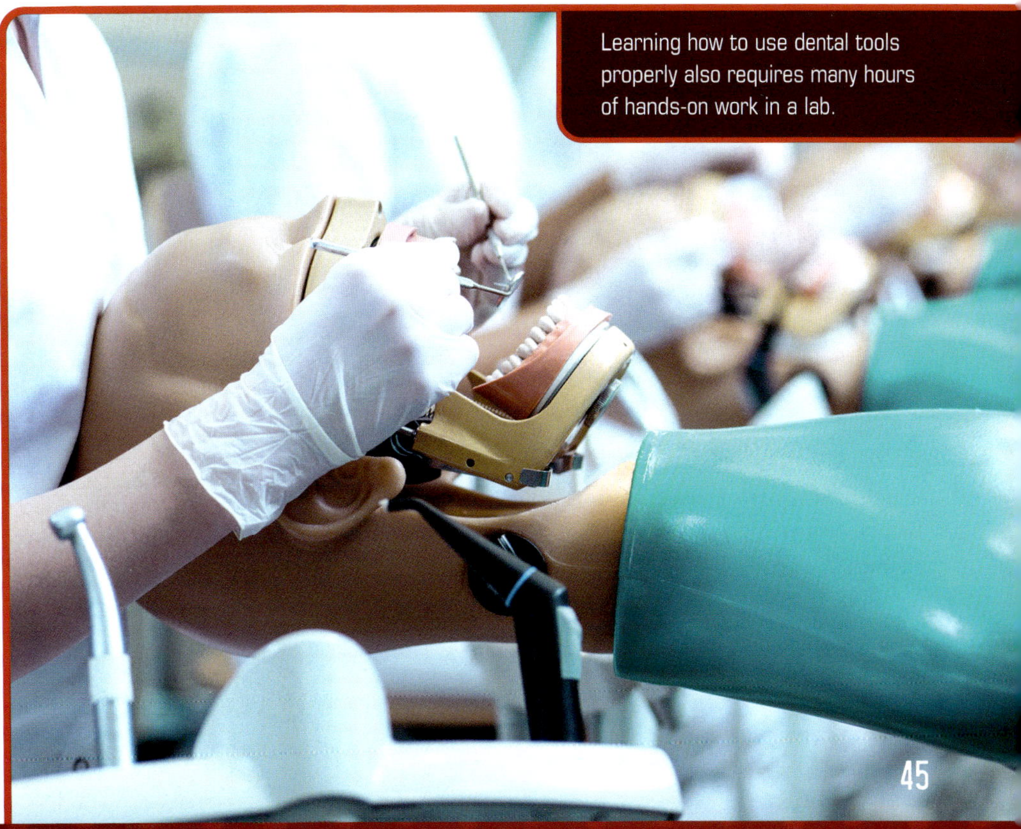

Learning how to use dental tools properly also requires many hours of hands-on work in a lab.

In the clinical portion of the program—the hands-on practice—the student performs services for real patients under the supervision of an instructor. Hygienist programs generally have their own clinics for this purpose. Often people in the community can schedule appointments at the training clinics and pay less than they would at a dental office. The services usually take longer because the students are learning. In addition to using the school's clinic, most programs require their students to take some of their clinical hours in a public health setting.

With an associate's degree or a certificate, a graduate is prepared to work in a private dental office. People who want to work in public health or pursue other career paths need to have a bachelor's or master's degree. Earning a bachelor's degree takes two additional years of study. Students in bachelor's programs take more classes in chemistry, health education, and counseling patients. They also have more hours of clinical practice. The extra training enables them to work in a community setting or as teachers or researchers.

MASTER'S DEGREE PROGRAMS

Master's degree programs are intended for dental hygienists who already hold a bachelor's degree and license. According to the American Dental Education Association (ADEA), less than 20 schools throughout the United States offer the Master of Science degree in dental hygiene or a related subject. Some of these programs are available online, others are on-campus, and some are hybrid. These programs have classes in research, leadership, education, and science.

With a master's degree, a hygienist can train other clinicians, lead clinics and other programs, and perform research. Graduates of master's degree programs often become managers or consultants.

DEGREE COMPLETION PROGRAMS

Most hygienists enter the field with a two-year degree or certificate. They may decide after working for a while that they want the skills and the opportunities a four-year degree offers. Hygienists with a license and an associate's degree or a certificate can go back to school and earn a bachelor's degree. They do so by enrolling in a degree completion program. There are a variety of programs to choose from. Some are offered partly or entirely online. They allow a hygienist to obtain a Bachelor of Science degree in dental hygiene, health science, or allied health.

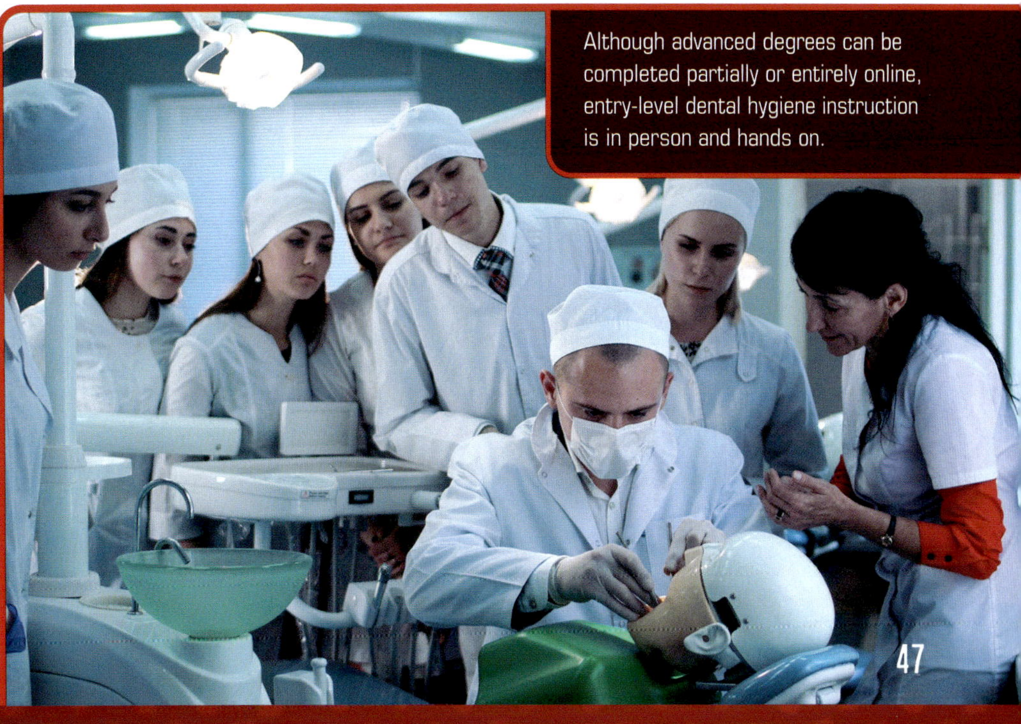

Although advanced degrees can be completed partially or entirely online, entry-level dental hygiene instruction is in person and hands on.

The National Board Dental Hygiene Examination (NBDHE) is the test prospective dental hygienists must pass to get their license. Here are some sample questions:

Fluoride is typically introduced in all of the following ways except by?

a. Drinking water
b. Vitamins
c. Injection
d. Toothpaste
e. Mouthwash

Gingivitis is considered controlled when?

a. The gums reach the crown.
b. No deep pockets appear in the gums
c. The gums appear firm
d. The plaque has been removed
e. There's no bleeding around the gums

A flat stone may be used to sharpen a curette by hand. The face of the curette should be at what angle to the stone?

a. 50–65 degrees
b. 75–85 degrees
c. 90–100 degrees
d. 100–110 degrees
e. 125–135 degrees

A dental carie is another name for a?

a. Dental instrument
b. The gum line
c. Cavity
d. Plaque build-up
e. Gingivitis

Which of the following is one of the main reasons for a root canal?

a. Tooth is cracked
b. The pulp can't be fixed
c. Gums are bleeding
d. A cavity is present
e. Enamel is worn off

Answers: C, E, D, C, B

Prospective dental hygienists need to possess a love of learning. Aside from their initial education and licensing exam, they'll need to complete continuing education programs throughout their career. They may also wish to complete a more advanced degree.

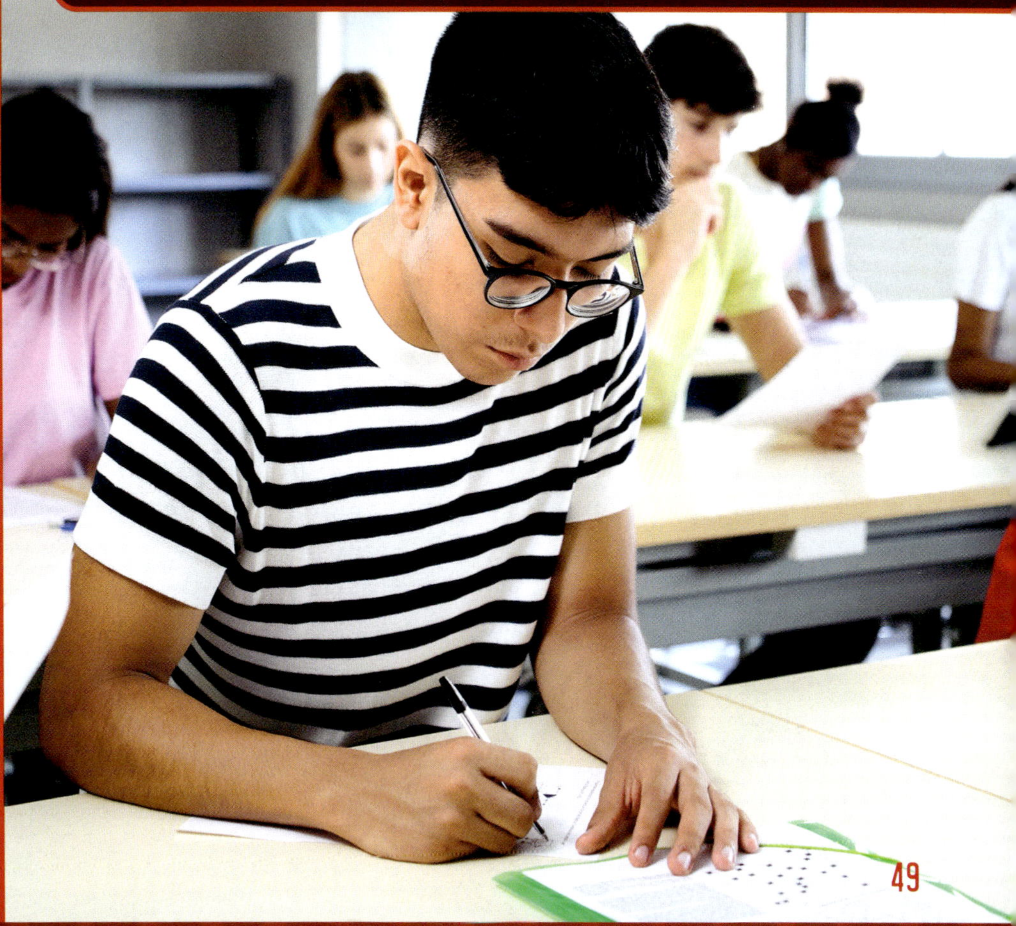

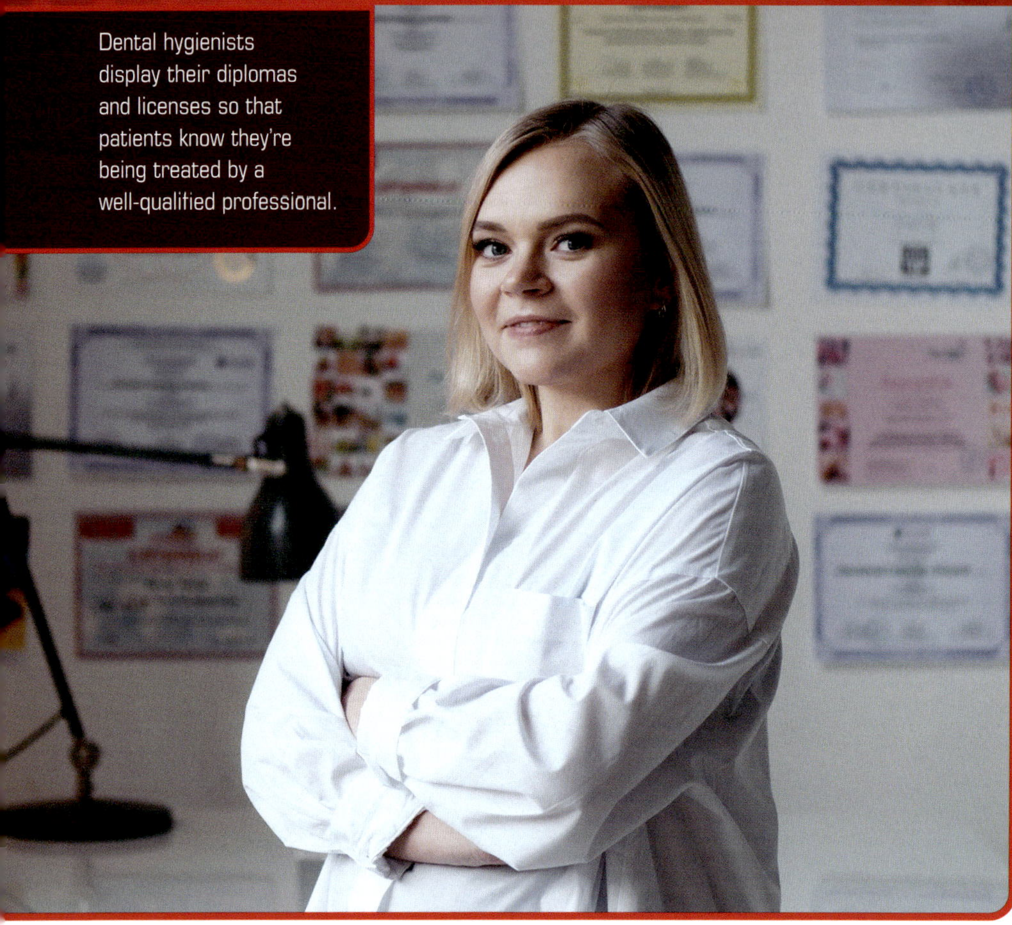

Dental hygienists display their diplomas and licenses so that patients know they're being treated by a well-qualified professional.

STATE LICENSE

Completing an educational program is a huge milestone. The next step is obtaining a license. Education gives dental hygienists knowledge and skills; a license proves the knowledge and skills are good. Each state has its own requirements for obtaining a license. A hygienist may move within a state without having to get another license. However, if they move out of state, they need to have a current license to apply for a new one in their new state of residence. The ADHA is working to make license more easily portable.

There are three steps to getting a license: graduation from an entry-level dental hygiene program and passing two exams. One exam tests knowledge, and the other tests skills. The test of knowledge is a written test. The National Board Dental Hygiene Examination (NBDHE) designed by the ADA is required for licensure in all 50 states. The NBDHE is a 7.5-hour test. It's divided into two parts. The first part asks 200 questions about basic science, oral health, hygienist practices, diseases of the mouth, dental materials, and other topics that hygienists should know. The second part gives scenarios that hygienists might encounter, and the test taker must make decisions about patients' condition or treatment. A grade of 75 is required to pass the exam.

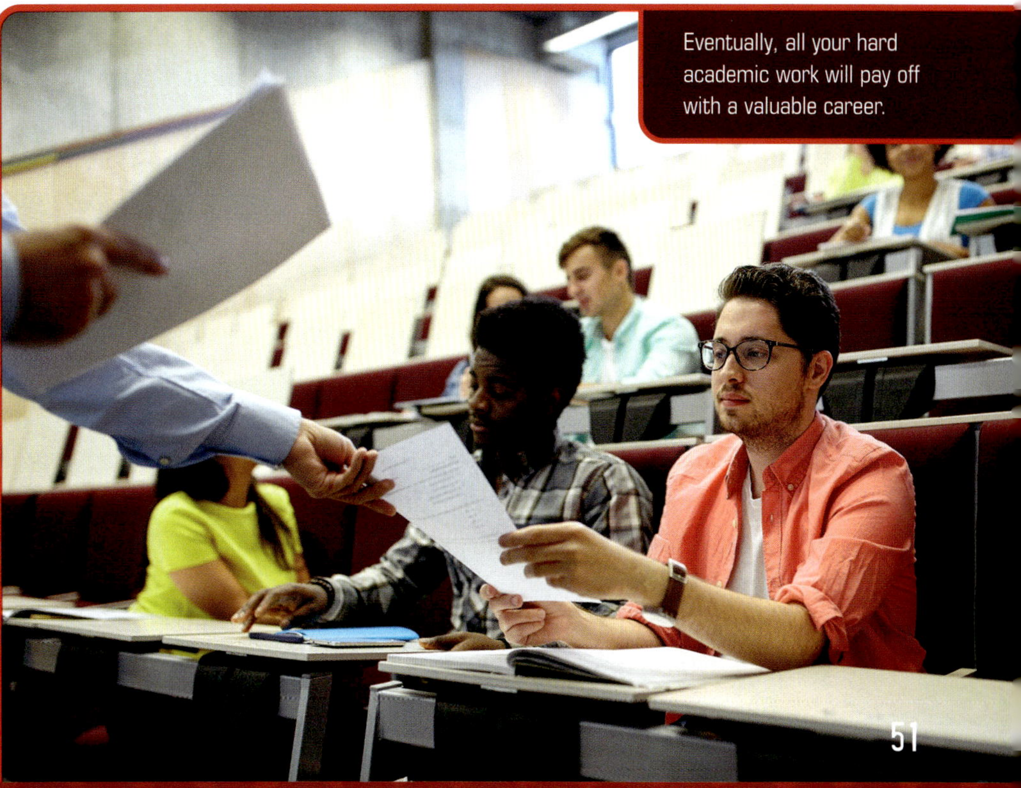

Eventually, all your hard academic work will pay off with a valuable career.

Hygienists need to demonstrate practical skills in order to earn their license.

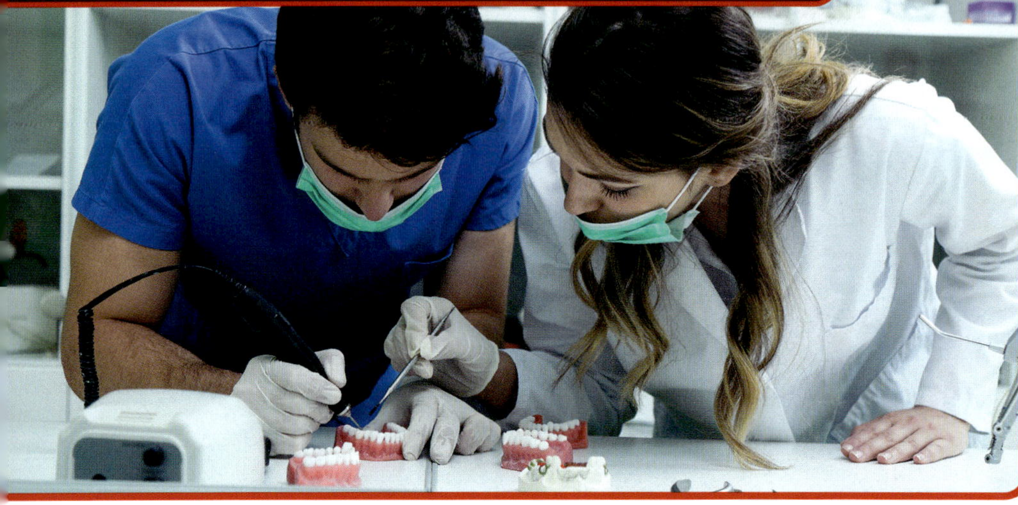

The test of skills—the clinical test—is a state test. Each state or group of states (region) has its own test. In the clinical test, test takers demonstrate their skills on real people. The candidate performs dental services on a real person and is critiqued by licensed dental professionals. States may have additional requirements for obtaining a license. Many require hygienists to be certified in CPR. Some give tests on the legal aspects of the profession. Most states also require hygienists to have continuing education to keep their licenses. They must have a certain number of hours of training every year or two to keep their knowledge and skills current.

When all the requirements are met, dental hygienists proudly use the letters RDH—Registered Dental Hygienist—after their names. These letters show that a person has completed at least two years of a very demanding training program and passed two long and difficult tests. They are now a registered dental hygienist. Their license will be proudly displayed on the wall in their treatment room.

ECO-FRIENDLY DENTISTRY

Like many other industries, dentistry now strives to be more eco-friendly. This can include things such as installing energy-efficient appliances and water efficient fixtures to save water, electricity, and ultimately money. It also includes practices such as recycling, and choosing products that are biodegradable or shipped in recycled packaging.

"Green dentistry" practices use digital records whenever possible. This reduces paper waste and space used for storage. Digital X-rays also help save space while using 75 percent less radiation than traditional X-ray systems. While new technologies can initially be expensive to install, they save money over time. Being known as an eco-friendly practice can also attract clients trying to live a more socially conscious lifestyle.

Today, many people are very conscious of how their actions impact the environment. They may go out of their way to choose a dental practice that is eco-friendly.

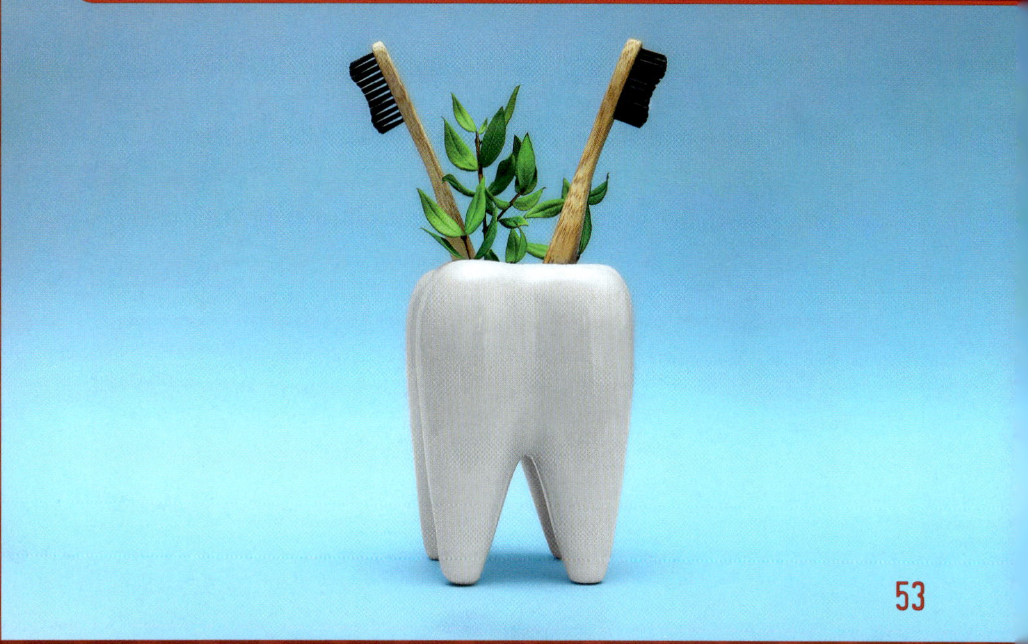

CHAPTER FIVE

A FLEXIBLE CAREER CHOICE

People have lots of reasons to choose dental hygiene as a career. They might want flexibility in their schedule instead of being tied to a 9-to-5 schedule. They want to work part-time or particular hours. Some love science and medicine and want to work in that field. Some choose the profession because dental hygienists make good money. Others like medicine or dentistry but want to go to school for only two years to start. Whatever the motivation, a lot of people select dental hygiene as a career.

The BLS reported there are more than 200,000 jobs for dental hygienists in the United States as of 2022. It expects another 16,000 jobs to open each year over the next decade. About half of all hygienists work part-time. Many have more than one job, combining part-time positions to work full days. A number of them work as clinicians and as teachers, researchers, or in other career paths.

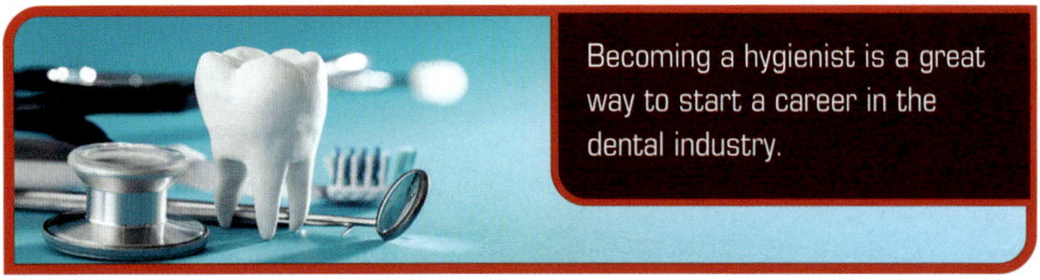

Becoming a hygienist is a great way to start a career in the dental industry.

A GROWING PROFESSION

The BLS predicts a faster-than-average growth rate in dental hygiene over the next decade. The large baby boomer generation is aging, adding to the elderly population requiring additional medical care. The rising costs of health insurance and medical care make people more conscious of preventative care. There are also community outreach programs designed to bring more health care to underserved populations. All these factors lead to a need for more dental hygienists in the future.

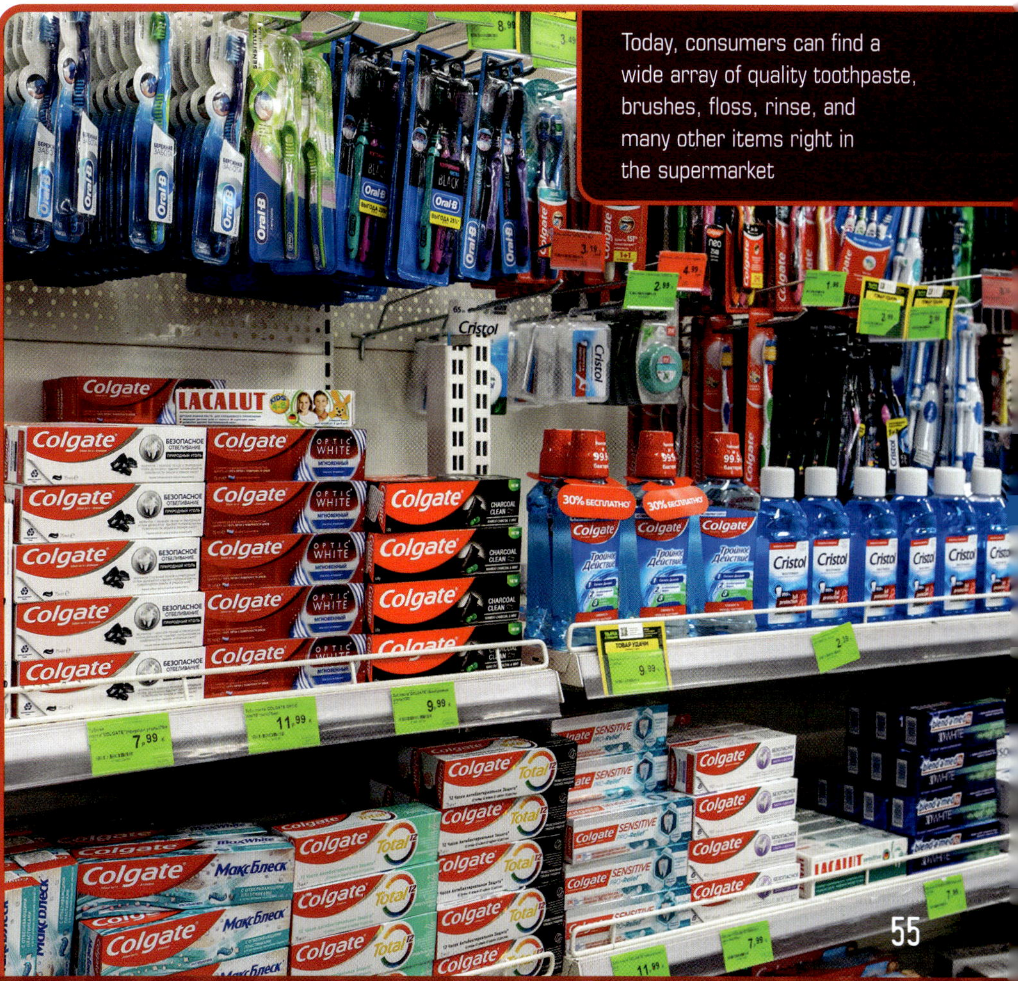

Today, consumers can find a wide array of quality toothpaste, brushes, floss, rinse, and many other items right in the supermarket

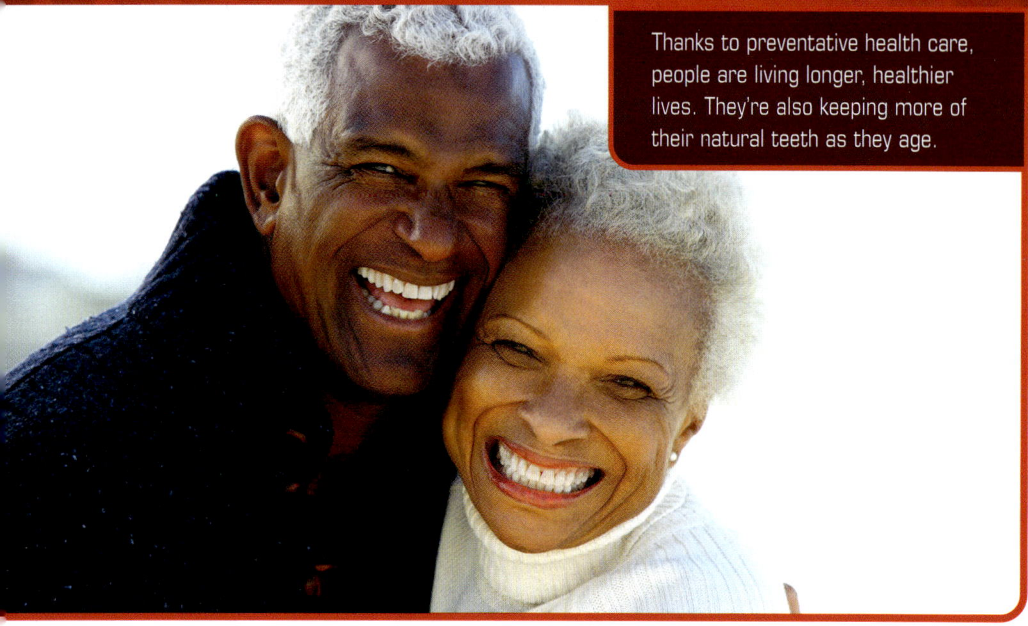

Thanks to preventative health care, people are living longer, healthier lives. They're also keeping more of their natural teeth as they age.

One reason the demand for hygienists is so high is that people are living longer and keeping their natural teeth longer than they used to. In years past, many people lost their teeth by the time they reached 60, 70, or 80 years of age. Most elderly people expected to have false teeth. Today, however, many people can expect to have most of their natural teeth all their lives.

The reason more people keep their teeth so long is that they understand the importance of preventive dental care. They were taught at a young age to take good care of their teeth. They are having their teeth cleaned twice each year. They are brushing and flossing properly. They have easy access to many products to take care of their teeth, and they are taking advantage of them. Insurance companies recognize that preventing tooth and gum problems saves money, so more companies offer better insurance. That means more people can afford the type of care dental hygienists offer.

New tools and materials are helping people practice better oral hygiene. Fluorides and dental sealants help prevent cavities. Some electric toothbrushes are timed to help people brush for the right amount of time. People can even buy water flossers and sonic toothbrushes for use at home. New types of flosses, brushes, and stimulators enable people to massage their gums easily. Flavored pastes encourage children to brush regularly. Modern radiographs and other equipment let dentists and hygienists detect and treat problems earlier. All these factors mean that more people have more teeth for more years . . . and more hygienists will be needed to help them care for those teeth.

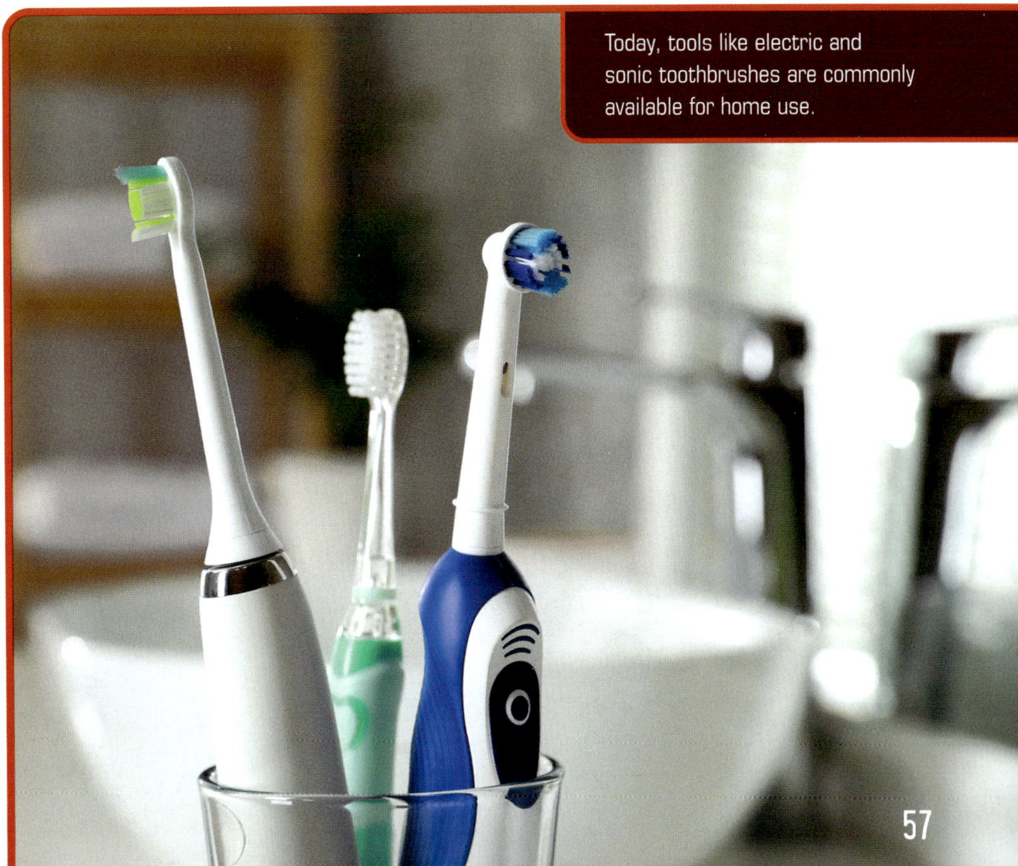

Today, tools like electric and sonic toothbrushes are commonly available for home use.

GEORGE WASHINGTON'S TEETH

Most people know that America's first president, George Washington, wore false teeth. This is true. What's not true is the legend that those teeth were made of wood. In fact, Washington's state-of-the-art dentures were made of lead, ivory, and real teeth. Some teeth were from animals. Others were human teeth he purchased from people he enslaved. Although the dentures were very sophisticated for the time, they didn't fit well and caused him pain. The teeth came loose and stained easily. They also pushed out his lips and made his face look odd.

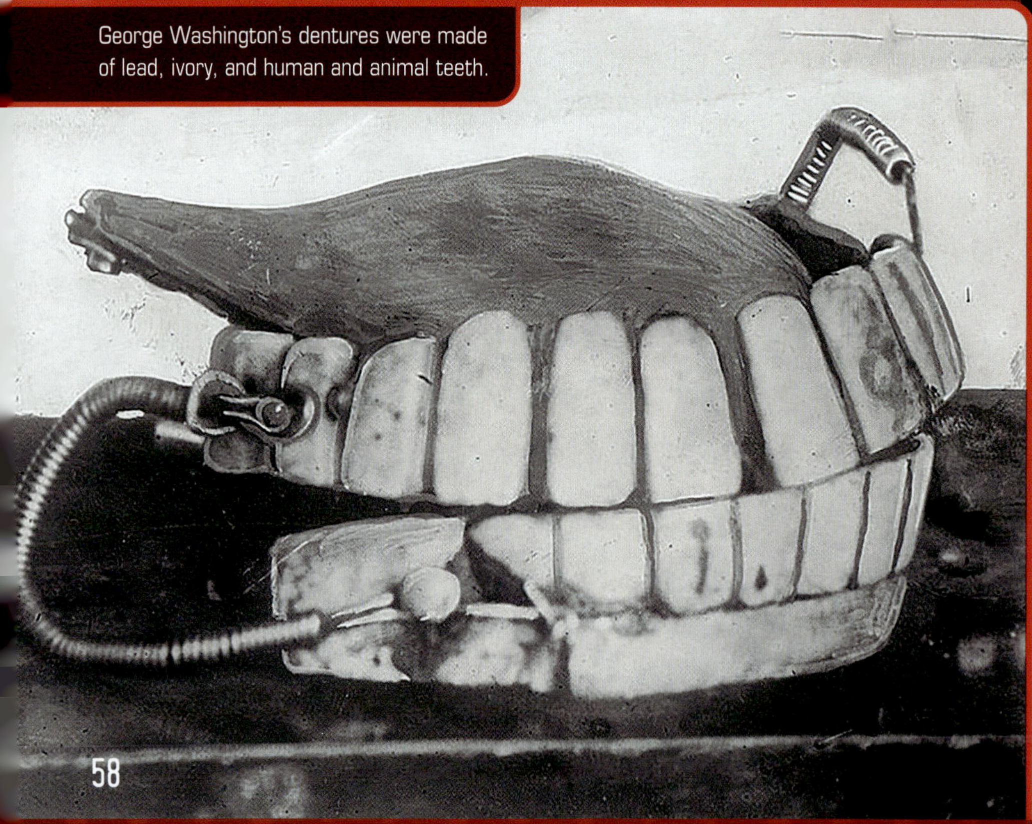

George Washington's dentures were made of lead, ivory, and human and animal teeth.

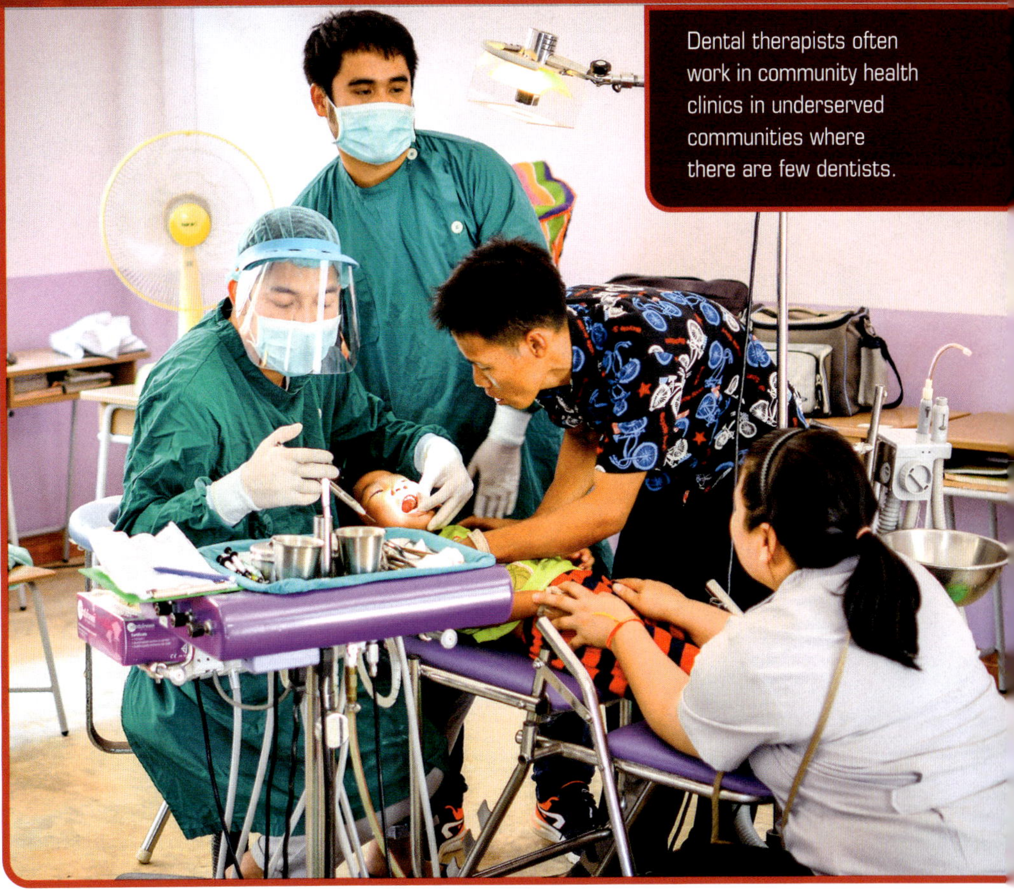

Dental therapists often work in community health clinics in underserved communities where there are few dentists.

KEEPING UP WITH THE DEMAND

According to the BLS, there are nearly 64,000 more hygienists than dentists. While the number of hygienists is rising, the number of dentists is not rising nearly as quickly. The number of dentists is not keeping pace with the number that is needed. In other words, demand for dentists is rising but supply is not going up at the same rate. One reason might be that becoming a dentist costs considerably more and takes longer than becoming a hygienist. People are increasingly conscious of the amount of student debt they take on. So, a less expensive education that produces a well-paying career is attractive.

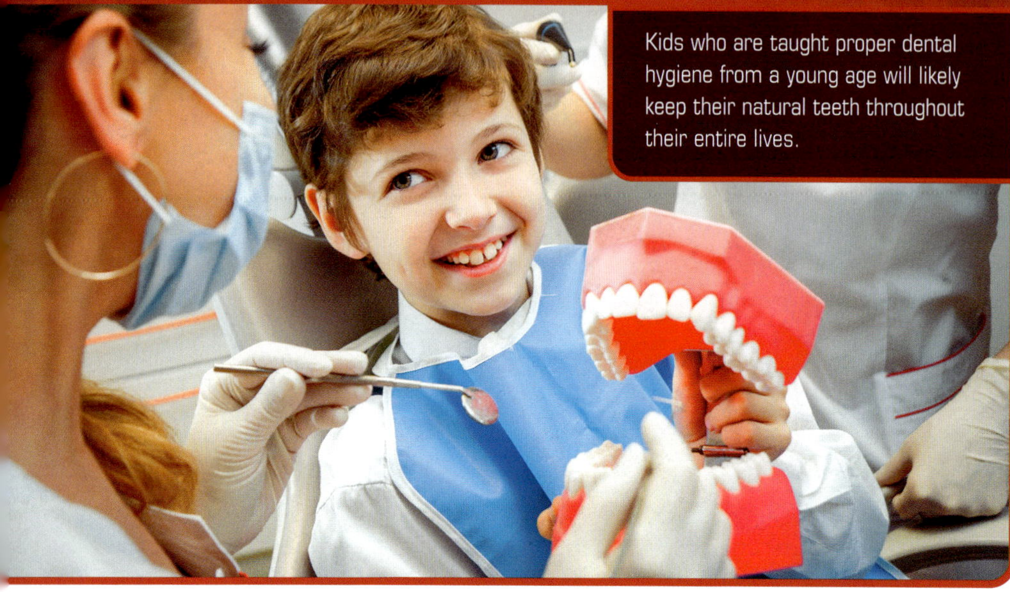

Kids who are taught proper dental hygiene from a young age will likely keep their natural teeth throughout their entire lives.

However, the workload of most dentists is increasing. Many dentists are asking their hygienists to perform some of the tasks the dentists normally do. They are having hygienists administer anesthesia and take out stitches the dentists put in. Hygienists sometimes put fillings in patients' teeth, and sometimes they smooth and polish crowns and bridges.

Some states permit hygienists to do these additional tasks, and some don't. If hygienists are to have more responsibilities, they will need more education. The solution is a new type of hygienist position that requires more education than a hygienist but less than a dentist. This new position has a couple of different titles: advanced dental hygiene practitioner (ADHP) or dental therapist (DT). The advanced hygienist or DT would have additional training and be able to perform more procedures than the registered hygienist. They may also be able to practice without the direct supervision of a dentist.

WHERE WOULD YOU LIKE TO WORK?

Advancing to become an ADHP or dental therapist is one possible career path for a dental hygienist. A similar path created by the drop in the supply of dentists is the registered dental hygienist in alternative practice (RDHAP). Currently, this position is offered only in California. Hygienists with this certification can work in nursing homes and other care facilities, schools, and homes of people who can't leave their houses. They can work in areas where there aren't enough dentists. They don't need a dentist's supervision, but if they serve one patient for more than 18 months, that patient has to get a prescription from a dentist authorizing more treatment. About 200 hygienists have RDHAP certificates. They must already hold an RDH license,

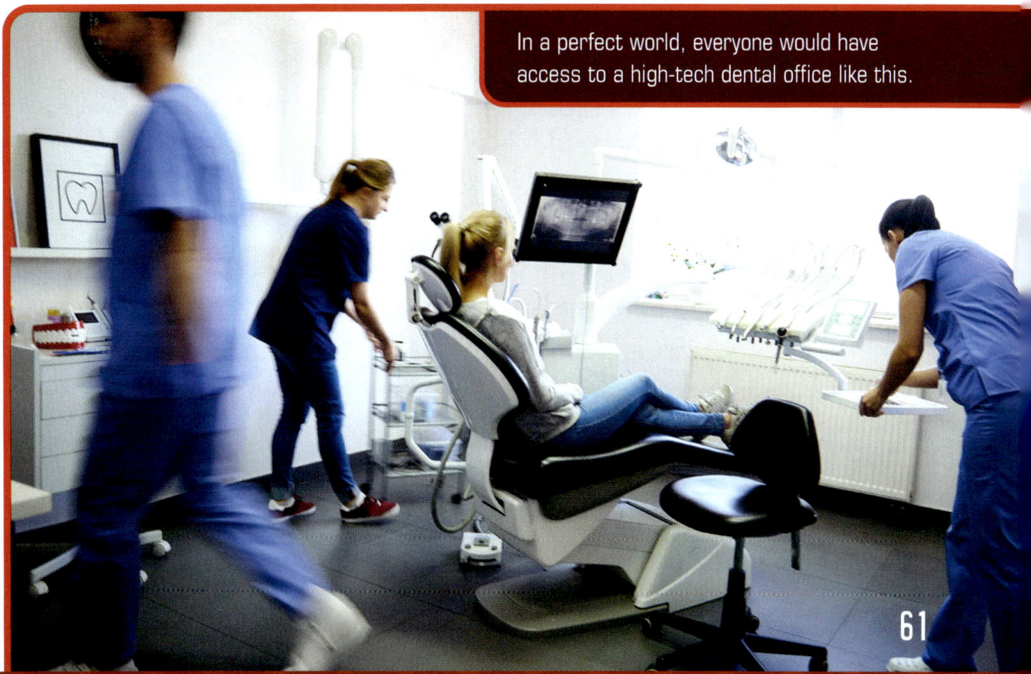

In a perfect world, everyone would have access to a high-tech dental office like this.

complete a bachelor of science degree, and an additional RDHAP course. RDHAPs are certified by the Dental Hygiene Board of California (DHBC).

Alternative practice, even in California, is rare. Most hygienists work in dental offices. Some work with general dentists, who see all kinds of patients, and some work with specialty dentists. The most common specialty practice for hygienists is periodontics, which deals with the gums. Another popular specialty is pediodontics, or children's dentistry. Some hygienists work with orthodontists, who straighten teeth and put on braces. Others prefer oral surgery, and still others work with cosmetic dentists, who are concerned with the appearance rather than the health of their patients' teeth and mouths.

All these career paths involve clinical practice. The non-clinical jobs described in Chapter 2 are also good careers for hygienists—in education, research, management, consulting, and forensics. The demand for hygienists in public health is growing. The shortage of dentists is most obvious in rural areas and places like Indian reservations. Many hygienists find a career in public health particularly rewarding for a number of reasons. Working in a community setting gives them the opportunity to do clinical work and education at the same time. It often requires less direct supervision. Public health hygienists usually work with a variety of people, both coworkers and patients. And they can often see that they are making a big difference in people's lives. Nearly half of all hygienists volunteer some of their time in public health, usually in schools or community health fairs.

PROS AND CONS

Of course, no career is perfect. There are pros and cons to every field of endeavor. One of the biggest benefits of a career in dental hygiene is its flexibility. Many mothers go into the profession because they want to work around their children's school schedules. They want to work only four or six hours a day, or they want to work evenings or weekends. The downside of the flexibility is that employees who work fewer than 40 hours every week may not receive benefits. They may not have health insurance, paid vacation, or paid time off when they are sick, or they may receive fewer benefits than someone who works full-time. Furthermore, hygienists who want full-time work sometimes have a hard time finding it. Some employers would rather pay two part-time hygienists instead of one full-time one because they don't have to pay as much in benefits. So hygienists might have to juggle more than one job.

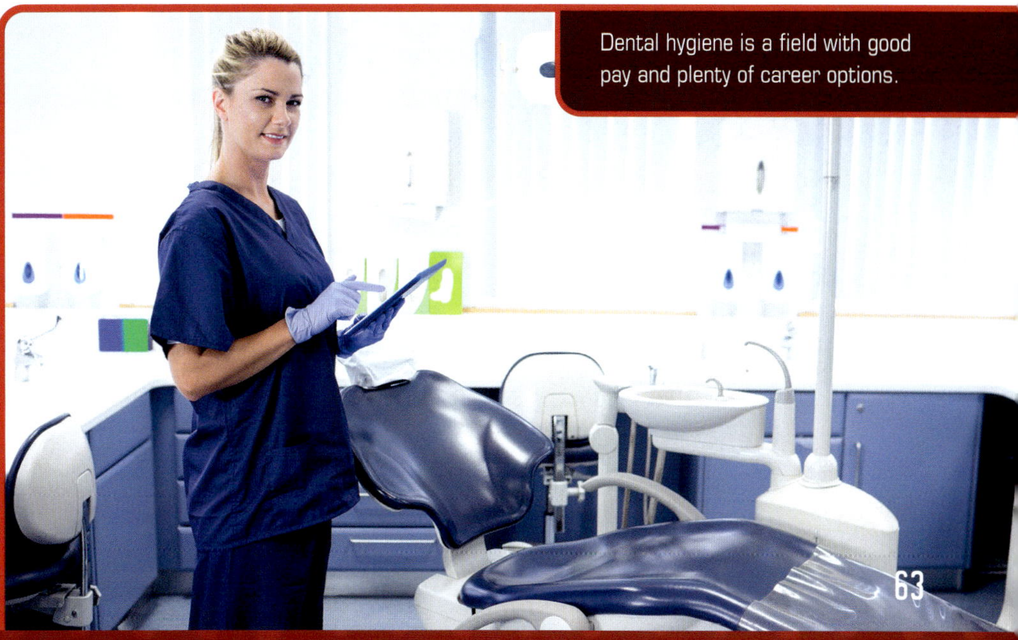

Dental hygiene is a field with good pay and plenty of career options.

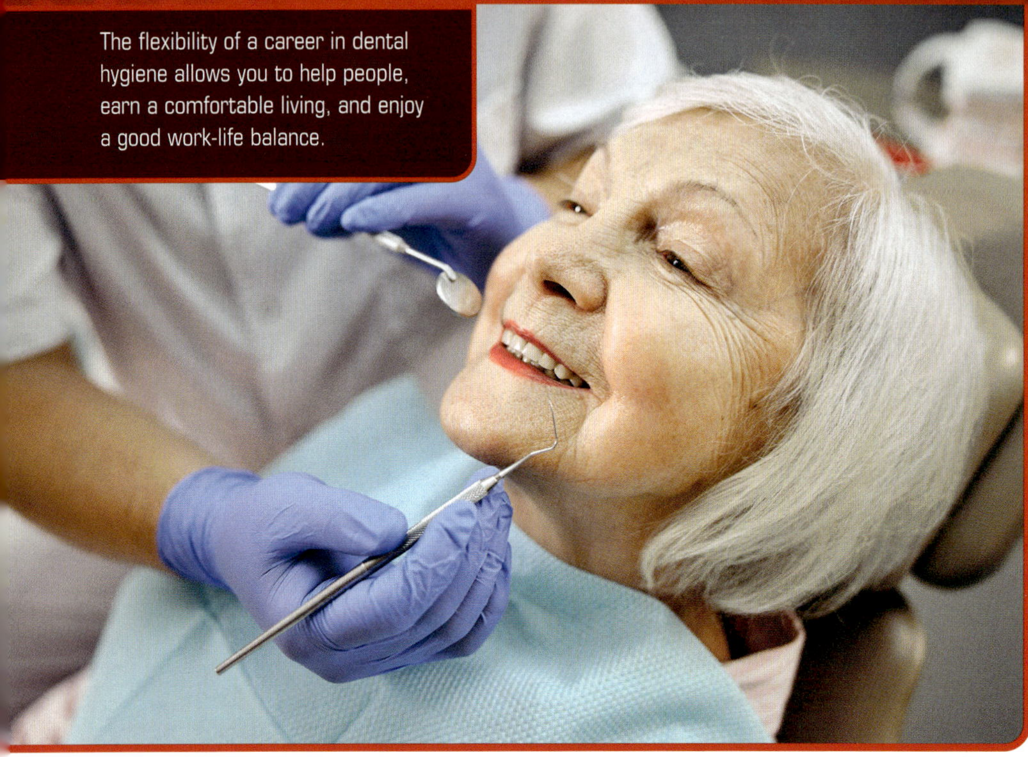

The flexibility of a career in dental hygiene allows you to help people, earn a comfortable living, and enjoy a good work-life balance.

One lure that draws many to this profession is its good pay. For more information about the average salary for a full-time dental hygienist, check out the BLS website (www.bls.gov). The income potential is especially high considering the short amount of time needed to qualify for the job. An entry-level position requires only a two-year degree. With the likelihood of high pay comes competition. Many people are trying to get into dental hygienist training programs, but there aren't enough programs for all the people who want them. Admission to dental hygiene programs is highly competitive. Candidates' grades might only be separated by tenths of a point, so researching schools, making sure to have the correct prerequisites, and making a good personal impression is very important. Getting the training to test for a license is becoming harder than it once was.

After people earn their RDH license, they might find competition in looking for a job, even though the need for hygienists is growing. The reason is that some areas of the country have lots of training programs—and therefore lots of graduates looking for work—and some have fewer. There is a high demand for dental professionals in rural areas where there aren't as many schools. A hygienist who decides to move to where the jobs are runs into a problem if the jobs are in a different state. An RDH with a license in one state must go through the clinical test in the second state to get a job there. Sometimes the second license has other requirements also, such as additional hours in training or practice.

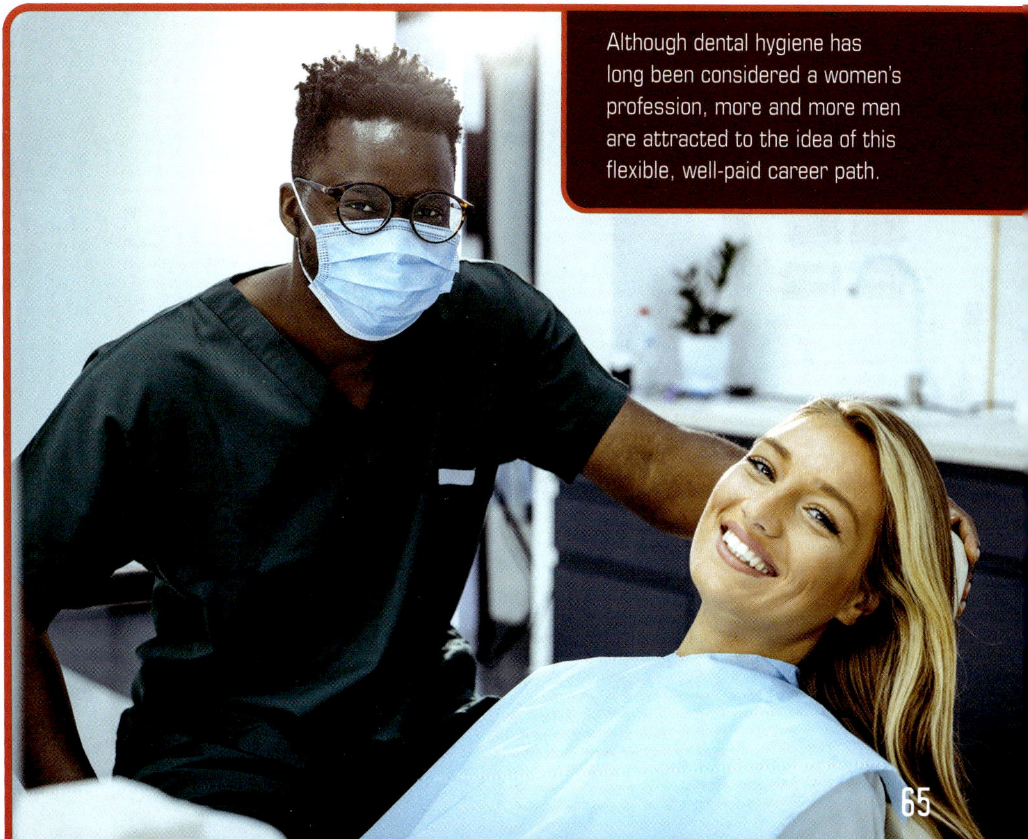

Although dental hygiene has long been considered a women's profession, more and more men are attracted to the idea of this flexible, well-paid career path.

Women especially find the flexibility and relatively high pay appealing. Dental hygiene is largely a female field; 98 percent of hygienists are women, according to the American Dental Hygienists' Association. A class of 30 might only have 3 or 4 male students. However, there's no reason a man wouldn't make a great hygienist. In fact, the few dentists who have hired male hygienists are quite pleased with them. Still, only a handful of men become hygienists. Similar to men becoming nurses, many are probably reluctant to enter a profession that most people see as women's work.

Despite the few minuses, all the pluses make a career as a dental hygienist a great choice. In light of industry growth, stability, salary, and job satisfaction, U.S. News and World Report rated dental hygienist as one of the best jobs in the country! Dental hygiene is ranked as the number 2 health care support job and number 35 in the 100 best jobs category.

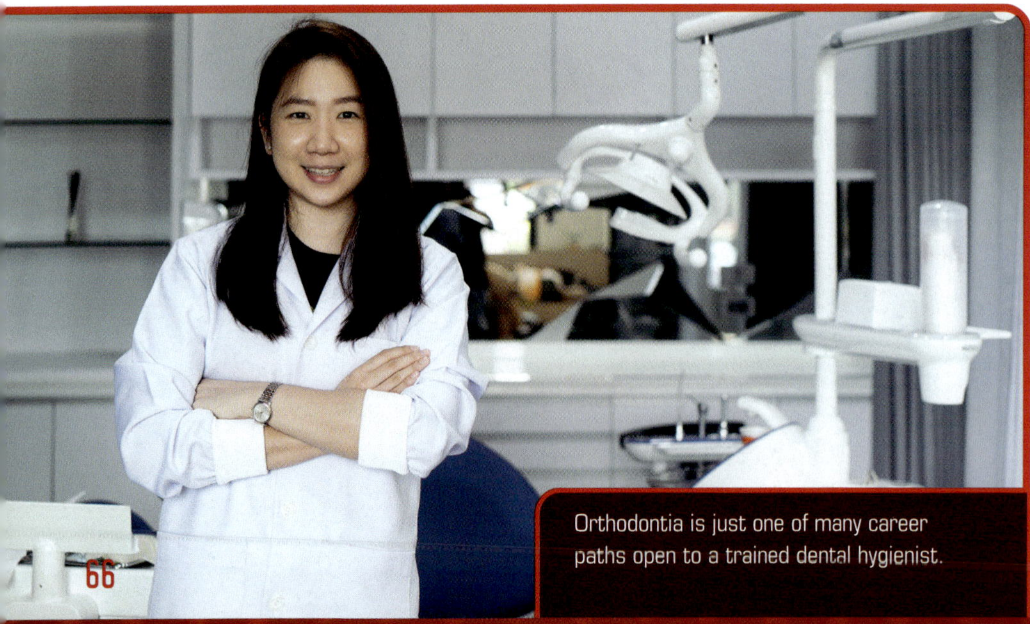

Orthodontia is just one of many career paths open to a trained dental hygienist.

ORTHODONTICS

Orthodontics is a dental specialty. Orthodontists treat teeth that have grown crooked or don't line up correctly when the patient bites. They use appliances the patient wears inside their mouth to correct the alignment of their teeth. This includes things such as braces and retainers, as well as the newer invisible alignment systems.

Although some patients are more interested in the cosmetic impact of having straight teeth, it's healthier if teeth line up correctly and all receive the same amount of wear when the patient chews.

Dental hygienists work in orthodontics practices. They adjust braces and appliances and talk to patients about oral hygiene. Brackets, braces, and wires are prime places for bacteria to collect, so it's even more important than usual for patients to understand and practice good oral hygiene.

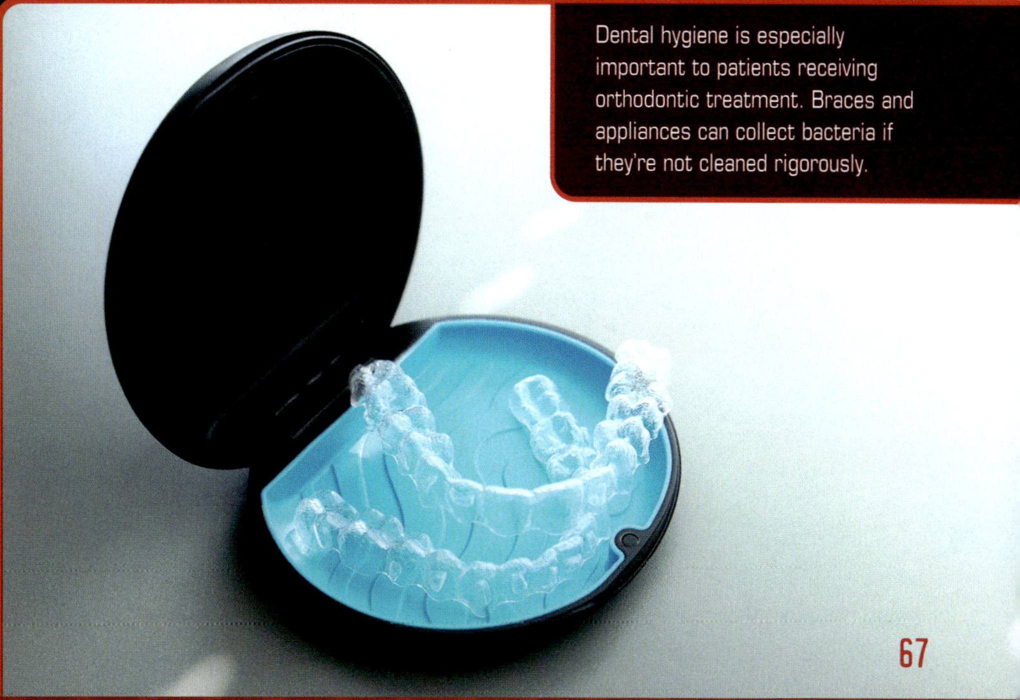

Dental hygiene is especially important to patients receiving orthodontic treatment. Braces and appliances can collect bacteria if they're not cleaned rigorously.

CHAPTER SIX

PLANNING YOUR CAREER

Like any big decision, a career in dental hygiene takes careful planning and assessment. A career in any form of dentistry requires specialized training. Before you commit to—and pay for—that training, you need to be sure dental hygiene is the right path for you. Does it suit your personality? Can your family reasonably afford the cost of schooling? And most importantly, will you be happy doing this every day for years?

The basic steps in pursuing a career in dental hygiene are the same as for achieving any important goal: assess your aptitude, gather all the information you can, develop a plan, and work your plan.

Start by gathering information. What schools are nearby? How much do they cost? How far are you willing or able to travel for school?

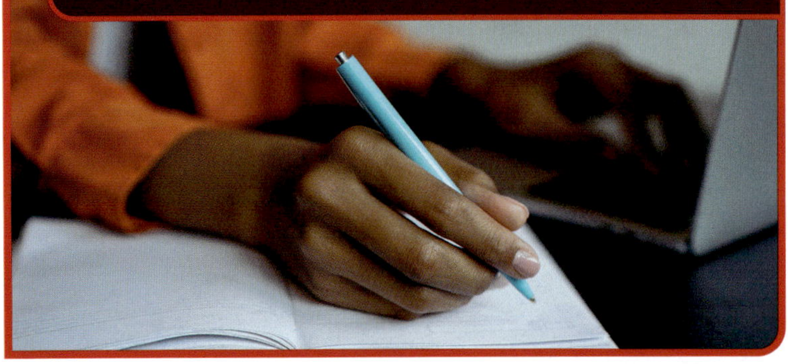

HAVE YOU GOT WHAT IT TAKES?

Assessing your aptitude means finding out if the job is something you would actually enjoy. You need to consider all the things dental hygienists do and decide if you're good at those things, and if that's what you really want to do. Do you like science and medicine? Does working on other people's teeth and mouths sound interesting to you? Are you comfortable with all kinds of people? With being very close to them? Can you work well both independently and as part of a team? Can you remain pleasant and upbeat, even if your patient doesn't want to follow your instructions?

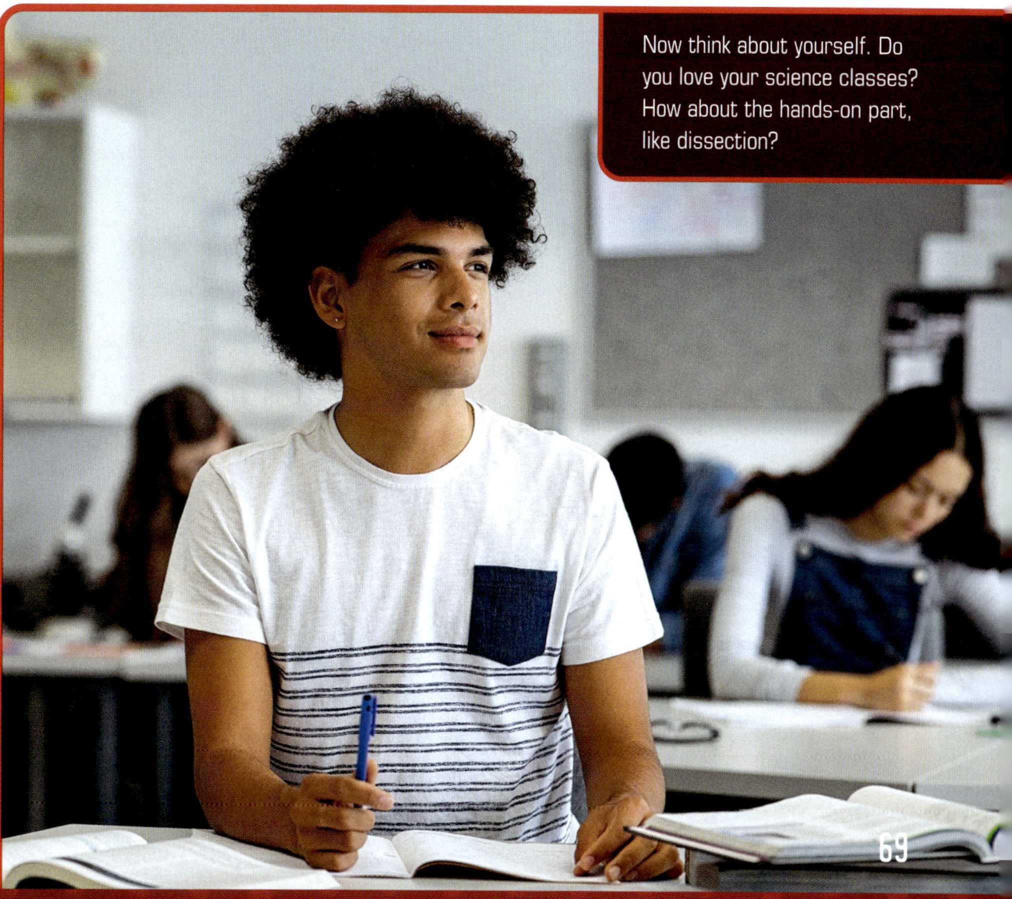

Now think about yourself. Do you love your science classes? How about the hands-on part, like dissection?

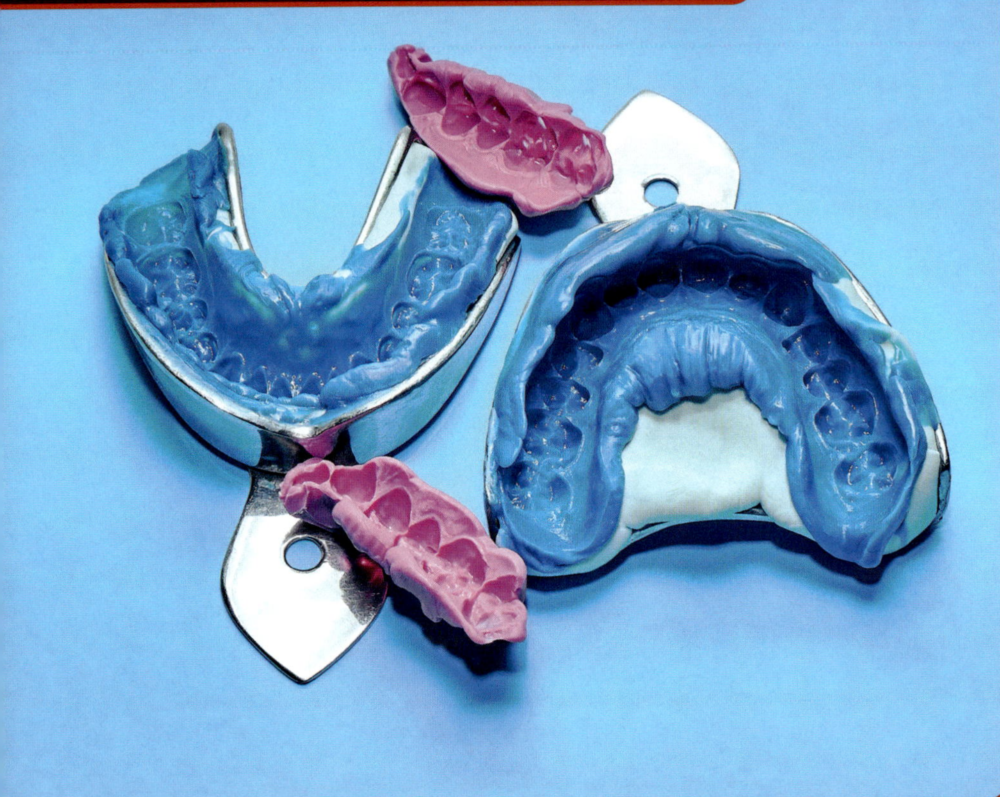

Dental hygienists take impressions of patients' teeth for different purposes. In orthodontics, it's a way to measure how well the teeth are straightening as treatment progresses.

Ask yourself if you have what it takes to do the job. Can you sit or stand in one spot for a period of time, or do you need to move around? Can you work carefully with your hands and fingers, or do you prefer large-muscle activities? Can you do close-up work without straining your eyes? Hygienists need good eyesight and manual dexterity. Do you pay attention to small details? A big part of the job is catching small imperfections before they turn into big cavities. Are you detail oriented? You'll need to keep careful records and organize lots of small, delicate tools.

High schools, community colleges, and technical schools often have career planning centers that can help you answer these questions. They have aptitude tests that let you know what kind of work is a good fit for your personality. These tests are usually pretty accurate at steering people toward jobs they are likely to enjoy. You don't just want a job you can handle; you want a career you will love.

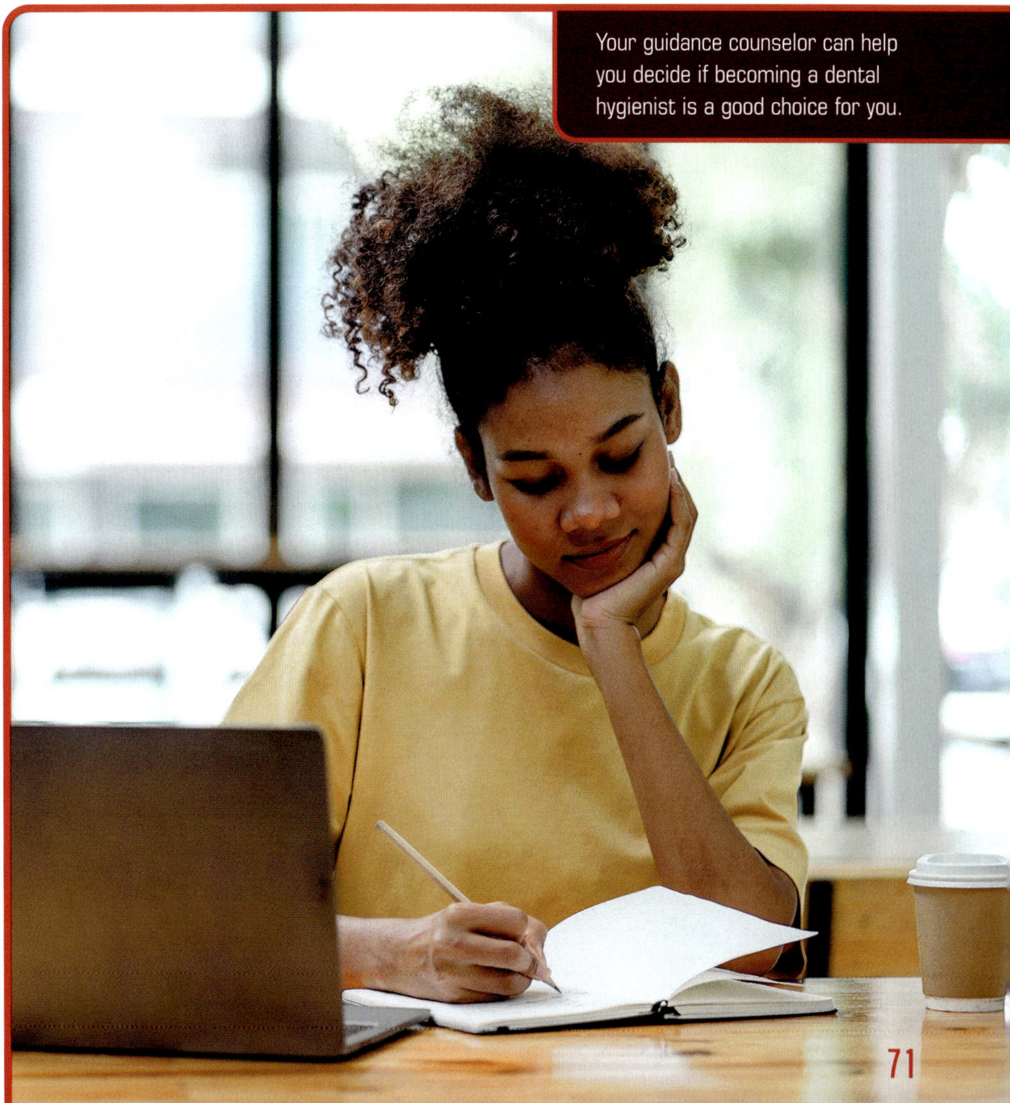

Your guidance counselor can help you decide if becoming a dental hygienist is a good choice for you.

GET THE FACTS

If dental hygiene sounds like a good career for you, find out everything you can about the job. Reading this book is a great start. Check out some of the books recommended at the end of this one. Talk to anyone you can find who works anywhere in the dental field. Talk with dentists, hygienists, dental assistants, and even receptionists in dental offices. Ask them what they like about their jobs and what they don't like. Ask if the job is what they thought it would be. If you can, talk with people in more than one office. Try to visit different kinds of practices. Is there an orthodontist's office nearby? An office that specializes in oral surgery? How about cosmetic dentistry? Would you like to work with kids? Try to get a feel for what it would be like to work in a dental office. Is the atmosphere calm? Stressful? Enthusiastic? Do the employees seem happy?

There is nothing like seeing the actual job. You may think you know what a hygienist does because of your experience at the dentist's office. But your hygienist probably works on patients with dental situations far different from yours. Moreover, the hygienist has many responsibilities before and after your visit. This can include things such as cleaning and recordkeeping. Watching a hygienist at work for a few hours or a few days will give you a better idea of what the job involves. Some professionals permit people to shadow them, to follow them around as they work and observe them. See if your school's career planning center can arrange for you to shadow a hygienist or a dentist. Or ask your own dentist or hygienist.

Some schools require prospective students to take the Health Occupations Aptitude Exam (HOAE) to be considered for admission to their allied health programs, including dental hygienist programs. The test consists of 305 questions that must be completed in 2 hours and 15 minutes. It includes five timed sections:

- academic aptitude
- spelling
- reading comprehension
- natural sciences
- vocational adjustment index

You can prepare for the first four sections as you would any other standardized test—by using an exam prep book, flashcards, or taking practice tests online. The vocational adjustment index is a series of questions designed to determine if you have the right personality traits for a career in healthcare.

When you're looking at dental hygiene programs, check to see if this test is required for admission.

Are there other kids in your class who are interested in careers in science or medicine? You can help each other study or maybe even look at schools together.

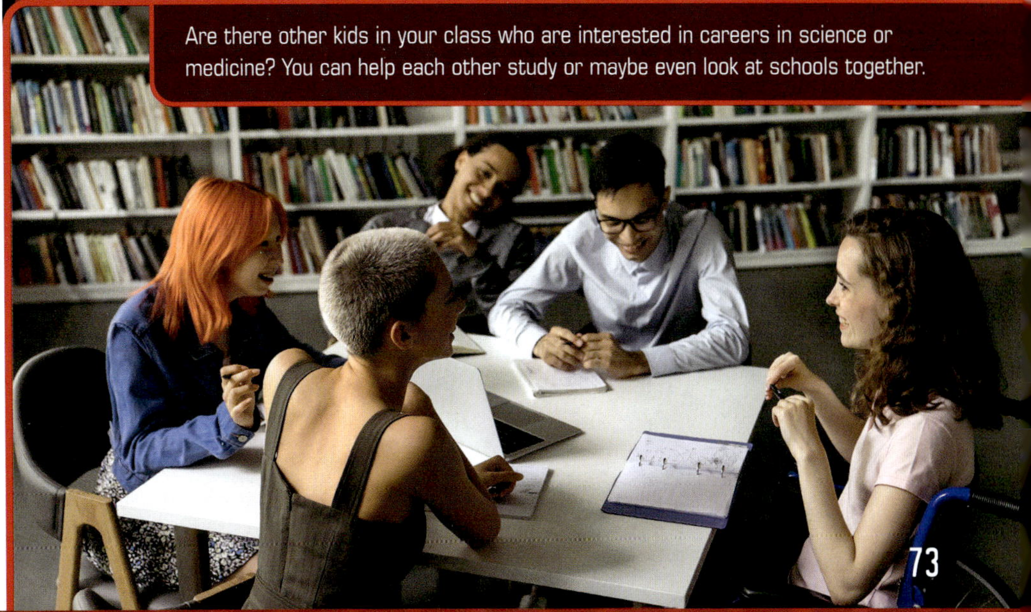

There are internships and volunteer opportunities available for high school students interested in allied health careers. Some organizations offer volunteer opportunities for people who aren't skilled but are interested in health careers. Usually, they are public health organizations that serve rural or low-income communities. The scope of activities is limited for unlicensed people, so you may simply assemble health care kits, pass out toothbrushes, clean and organize equipment, or entertain children as they wait for dental checkups. But you will be working alongside health care professionals, and that will give you a good feel for public health dentistry.

Working with dental professionals—in any capacity—is a great way to decide if it's the right industry for you.

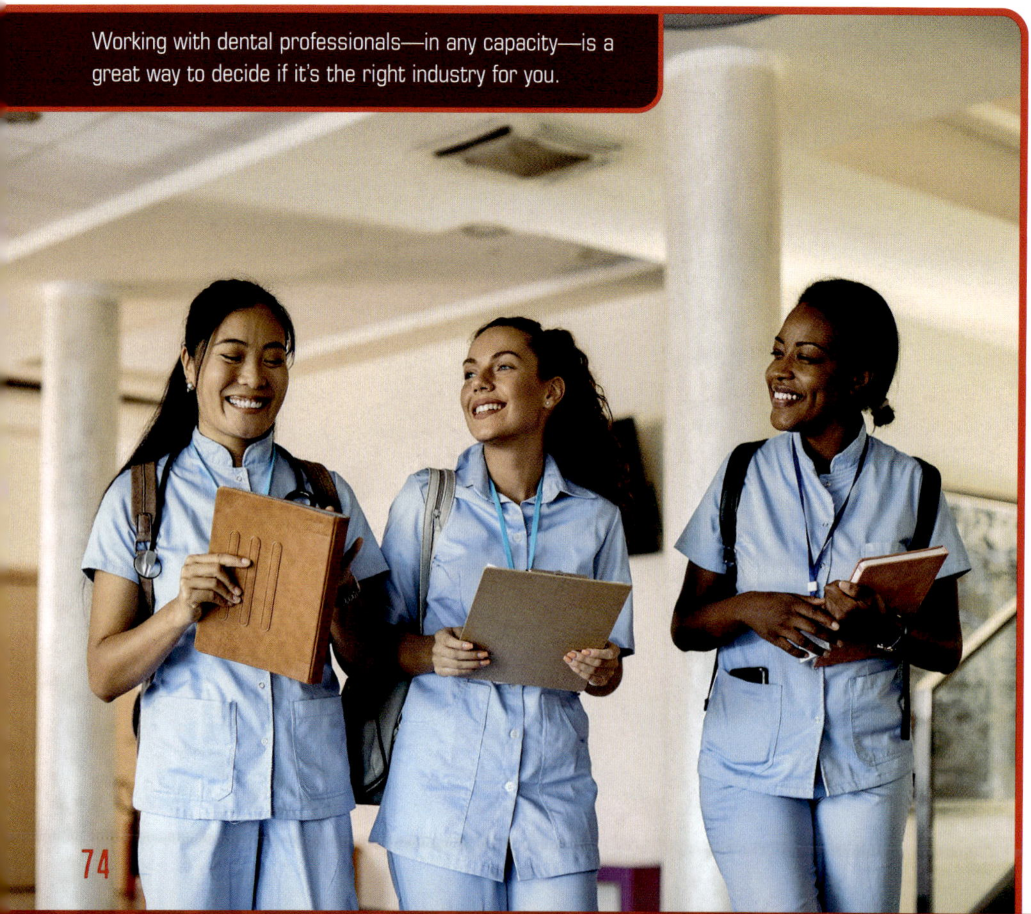

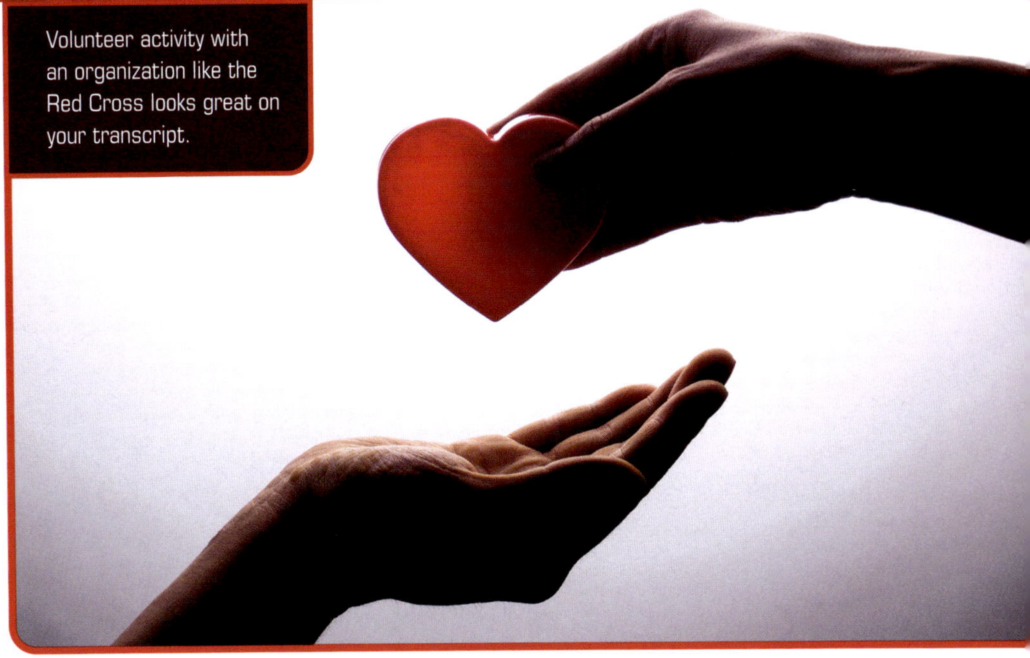

Volunteer activity with an organization like the Red Cross looks great on your transcript.

The Red Cross uses volunteers at blood drives, called blood donor ambassadors. These people don't perform medical services, but welcome donors, provide information and help them get registered. The Red Cross also trains volunteers for disaster relief. Activities such as these will give you some experience that will make you stand out when you apply for admission to a hygienist training program. If the schools in your area are hard to get into, your hands-on experience may give you an edge over other applicants.

Some schools offer summer intensives for kids interested in medical careers. Others have programs for kids from underrepresented or low-income communities. You need to research what's available where you live. Your guidance counselor should be able to help. The more "extras" you can put on your application, the more attractive you'll be to the admissions department.

THE FINAL FRONTIER

For all the flexibility offered by a career in dental hygienics, there's one place no dentist—or dental hygienist—has boldly gone. That place is space. There are good reasons for this. If you've ever read or watched *Hidden Figures* or *Apollo 13*, you know that it takes enormous amounts of energy and precise calculations to launch a spacecraft beyond earth's atmosphere. Every last gram of weight must be carefully considered. There simply is no room to send things "just in case."

Instead, what NASA and other space agencies do is make sure candidates for space flight have excellent dental health. This is to prevent an astronaut needing dental treatment while in space. Astronauts fall into three categories of dental health:

- Class I astronauts have good oral health and aren't expected to require dental treatment or evaluation for the next 12 months.
- Class II astronauts have some oral conditions that, if left untreated, aren't expected to result in a dental emergency within a 12-month period.
- Class III astronauts have an oral condition that, if left untreated, is expected to result in a dental emergency within a 12-month period.

These precautions are taken because the changes in pressure during space flight could cause pain in untreated cavities. The vibrations and g-force associated with launch are strong enough to vibrate fillings, crowns, or bridgework that have any flaws.

As space missions become longer, new means of dental care have evolved. Astronauts brush their teeth in zero gravity with toothpaste designed to be swallowed, instead of spit out. On the International Space Station, there are two regular astronauts called crew medical officers (CMO). They've passed special training to treat medical emergencies, including some dental emergencies. Their training is about the same as a paramedic, and they're supported by a medical team on earth.

Today, space agencies are planning missions to Mars that would take years. Scientists and doctors are thinking about what will be needed to provide for dental care on such a long mission.

As space missions become longer, it's necessary to devise ways to provide medical care to astronauts. Who knows? Maybe you could be the first dental hygienist in space!

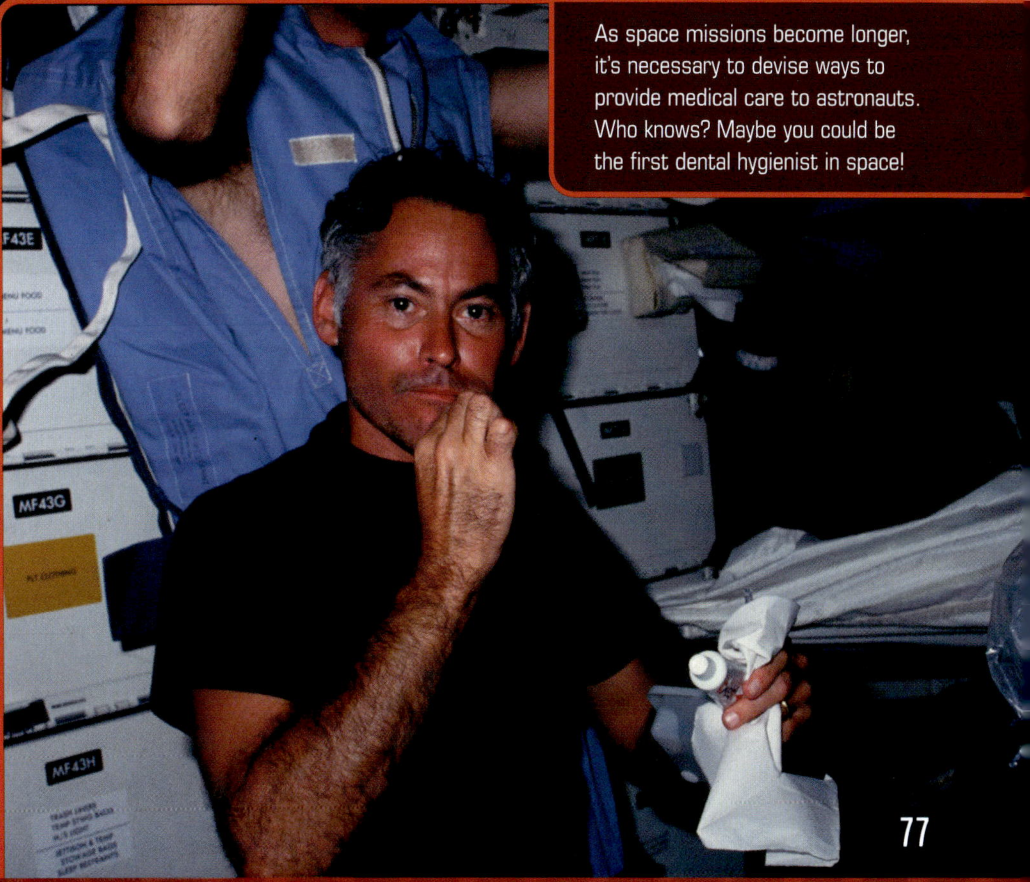

PLAN YOUR STRATEGY

One of the most important pieces of information you need to gather is what possibilities for training are available to you. What education programs are in your area? How much do they cost? What does it take to get into them?

Dental hygiene programs look at high school grade point average (GPA). You must have at least a C average, and the higher the average, the better. You will need to have courses in math, biology, chemistry, and English—and good grades in those classes. Programs also consider scores on college entrance tests such as the SAT. Again, the higher the score, the better your chances.

Usually, you must have some college before you will be accepted into a hygienist training program. Most programs want you to have about 40 college units of chemistry, English, speech, psychology, and sociology. They look at your GPA in those classes and may pay special attention to your grades in the science classes. Core credits such as these can usually be taken at a community college or a local state university campus, both of which cost considerably less than a private college. However, you need to be sure you're taking the correct prerequisites for the dental hygienist program you're interested in, as they do vary between schools.

You'll need to sit down with your folks and have a serious talk about money. How much can your family reasonably afford? How much student debt are you willing to take on? If you can train locally, it can reduce the cost of your education by thousands of dollars. If money is truly an obstacle for you, you may qualify for Job Corps' Dental Assistant program, which is free of charge to qualified individuals. You'd graduate with a well-paying career that would put you in a good position to go on to become a hygienist. Many training programs require applicants to take the Health Occupations Aptitude Exam (HOAE) before they're accepted into the program. Others may require an interview. Do your research, as each school has different requirements.

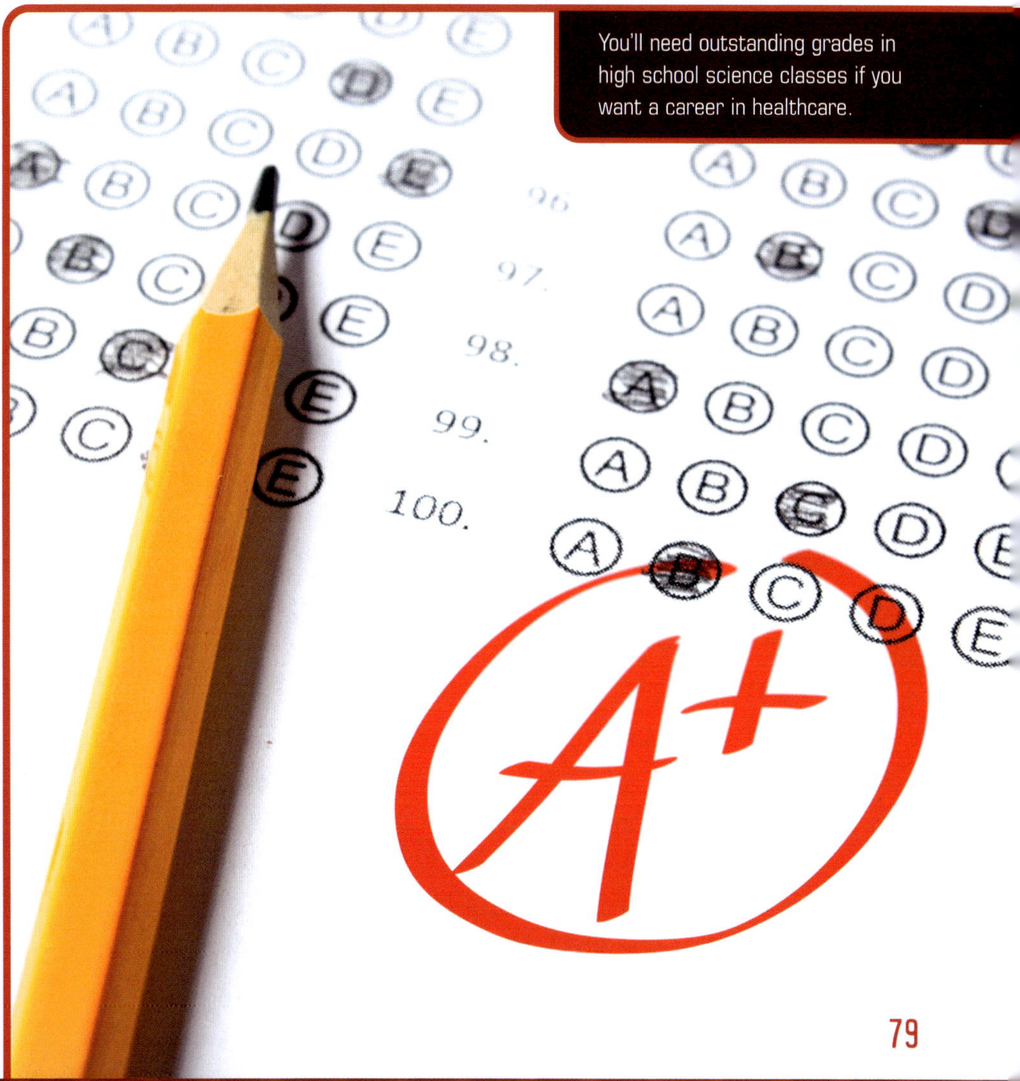

You'll need outstanding grades in high school science classes if you want a career in healthcare.

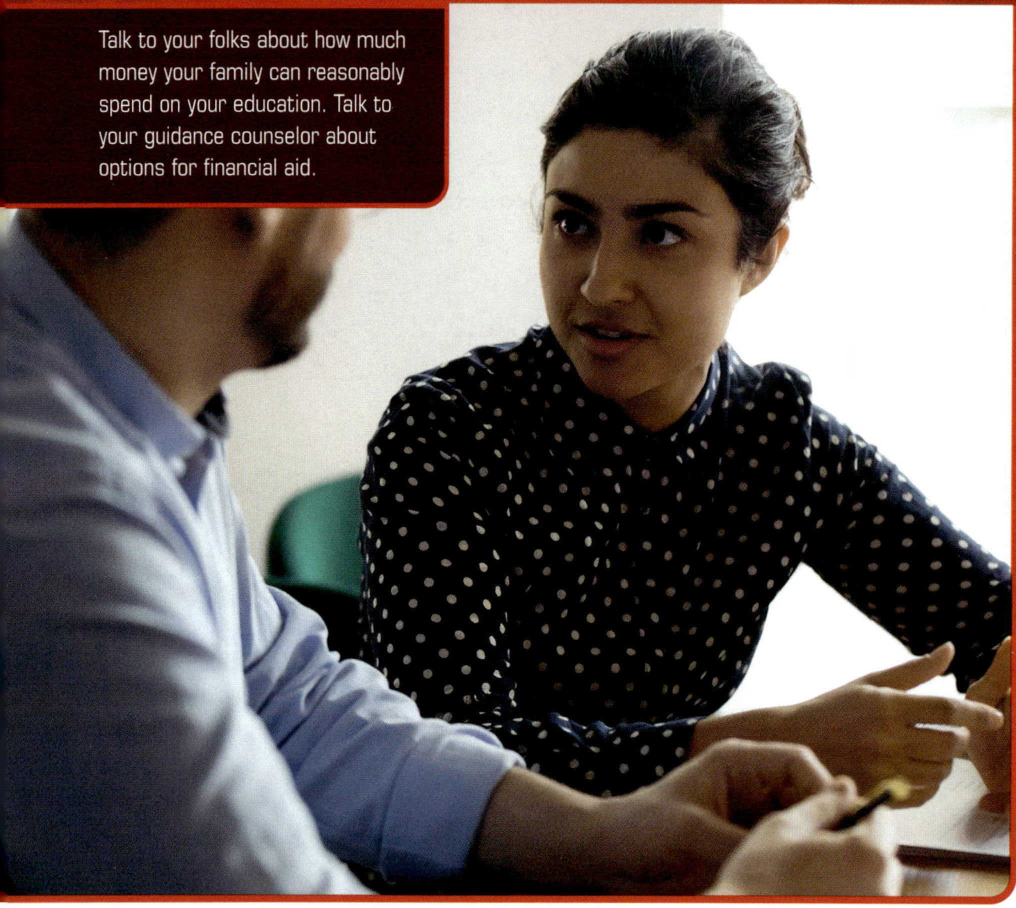

Talk to your folks about how much money your family can reasonably spend on your education. Talk to your guidance counselor about options for financial aid.

BEGIN YOUR JOURNEY

Now it's time to start your career journey. Your guidance counselor can be one of your strongest allies. They're your go-to person for information about scholarships and financial aid. They're your source for classes and extracurriculars that can make you stand out. Does your school offer honors or AP science classes? Take them. Is there a science club that would look good on your transcript? Join it. How about summer programs in science or healthcare? Find out if it's something you can afford or if you qualify for financial assistance.

Talk to dental professionals in your area. Find out where they went to school and if they recommend the program. Narrow down your choice of schools to make sure you're taking the correct prerequisites. Find out which standardized tests are required for entrance and plan your exam prep. See if there's any kind of summer job available in a local dental or medical office. Even if it's just basic clerical work, you'll still have the experience of being in a medical office on a daily basis.

There are a lot of steps to becoming a registered dental hygienist, but there's a satisfying career waiting at the end of the path!

Think seriously about how much student debt you can incur and whether you'll be able to hold a job and keep your grades up.

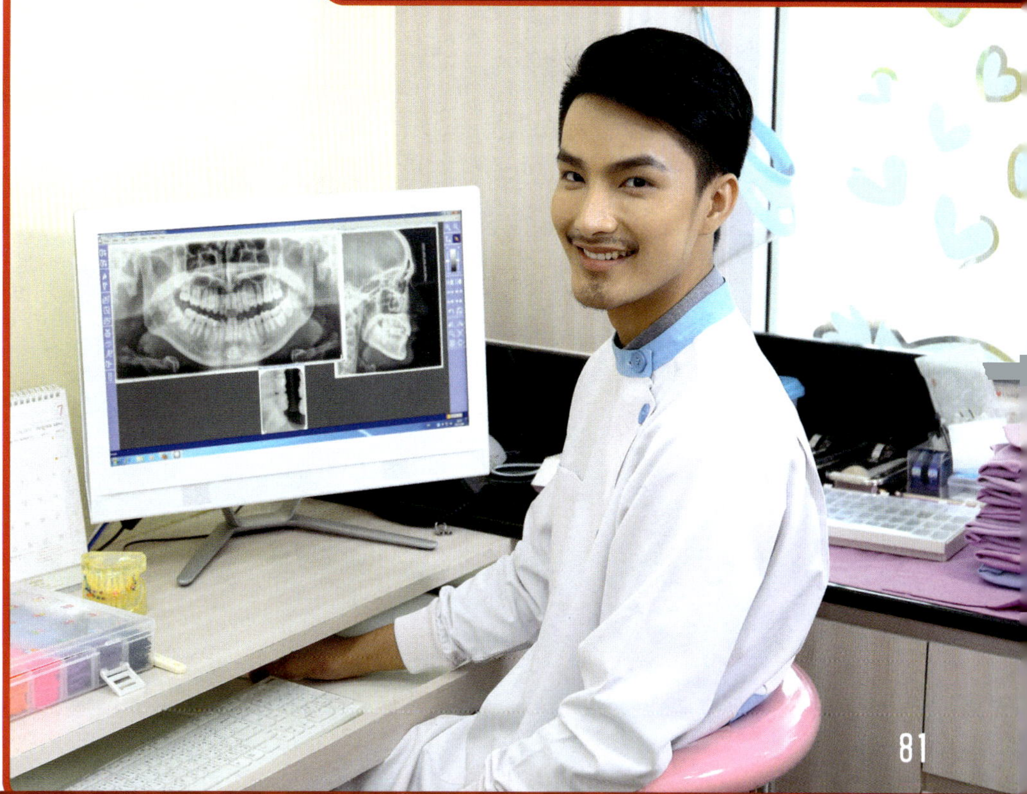

10 GREAT QUESTIONS TO ASK A DENTAL HYGIENIST

Here are some questions you can ask a dental hygienist.

1. What kind of degree do you have?
2. Do you think you'd like to go back to school to complete a higher degree?
3. How often do you have to take continuing education classes to maintain your license?
4. Are there any magazines or blogs you recommend?
5. What can I do to prepare for a career in dental hygiene while I'm still in high school?
6. Do you work full time or part time?
7. Have you ever worked someplace other than a dentist's office?
8. Is there a specialty you're interested in?
9. Do you belong to any professional organizations?
10. Is there anything you wish someone had told you when you first considered this career?

What other questions can you think of?

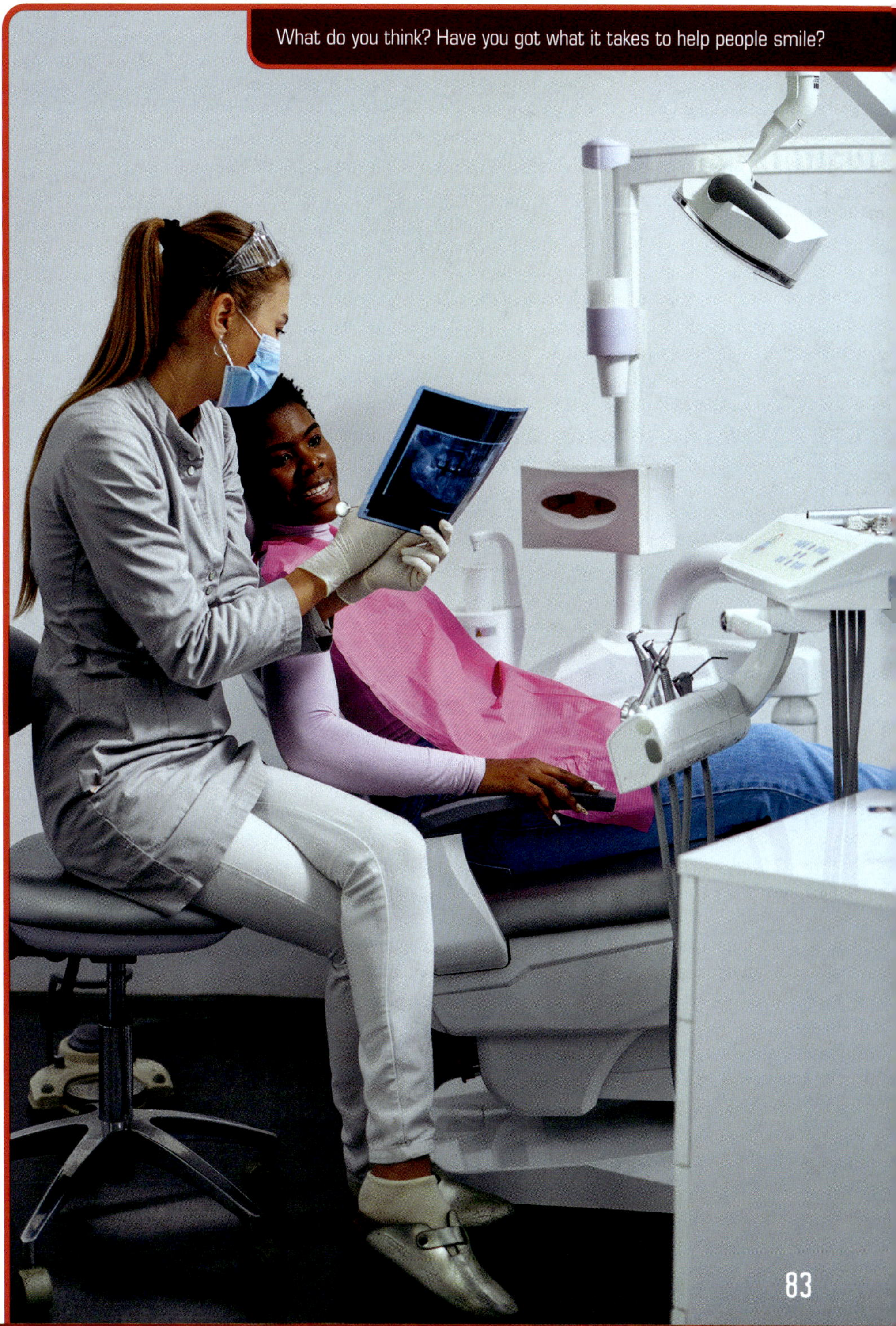

What do you think? Have you got what it takes to help people smile?

GLOSSARY

accredited: Authorized, or given approval, by a recognized organization.

advocate: A person who helps someone with less power gain the ability to accomplish something specific; a person who publicly supports or recommends a particular cause or policy.

anatomy: The science of the shape and structure of living beings or parts of living beings.

anesthetic: A substance such as a drug that is used in medical or surgical procedures to induce insensitivity to pain.

autoclave: Equipment that sterilizes items using pressurized steam.

calculus: Also called tartar, a hard deposit that forms on teeth. It is composed of plaque and minerals, especially calcium.

clinician: A person who practices one of the healing arts.

CPR: Cardiopulmonary resuscitation, an emergency procedure used to help revive a person whose heartbeat and breathing have stopped.

curette: A scaler with a rounded tip used for scaling below the gum line.

fluoride: A compound that contains fluorine, a natural element that inhibits tooth decay.

GED: General Educational Development, also commonly referred to as General Education Diploma or General Equivalency Diploma, a credential earned by a person who did not graduate from high school that certifies that the person has passed tests showing that he or she has the same academic skills as someone who graduated from an American or Canadian high school.

periodontal: Having to do with gums.

plaque: A soft, sticky film that builds up on teeth. It is composed of food, bacteria, and other substances that occur naturally in the mouth.

RDH: Registered dental hygienist, a certification given by the American Dental Hygienist Association showing that a person has completed all its requirements for practicing dental hygiene.

RDHAP: Registered dental hygienist in alternative practice, a certification offered in California that allows a hygienist to practice in certain settings without the supervision of a dentist. root planing: A dental procedure in which the surfaces of the tooth root are smoothed.

sanitize: To make clean; to free of bacteria and other germs.

scaler: An instrument used for scraping deposits from teeth.

tartar: Also called calculus, a hard deposit that forms on teeth. It is composed of plaque and minerals, especially calcium.

therapeutic: Designed to heal.

FOR MORE INFORMATION

AMERICAN ACADEMY OF PEDIATRIC DENTISTRY (AAPD)

211 East Chicago Avenue
Suite 1600
Chicago, IL 60611-2637
(312) 337-2169
Website: www.aapd.org
Facebook: @AmericanAcademyofPediatricDentistry
Instagram: @aapediatricdentistry
AAPD is a professional organization for dental professionals who work in the field of children's oral health.

AMERICAN DENTAL ASSOCIATION (ADA)

211 East Chicago Avenue
Chicago, IL 60611-2678
(312) 440-2500
Website: www.ada.org
Facebook and Instagram: AmericanDentalAssociation
The ADA is the organization that accredits dental professionals, policies, and products.

AMERICAN DENTAL EDUCATION ASSOCIATION (ADEA)

655 K Street, NW
Suite 800
Washington, D.C. 20001
(202) 289-7201
Website: www.adea.org
Facebook and Instagram: @ADEAweb
The ADEA is "The Voice of Dental Education" in the US. Their website contains a wealth of information for students of various dental disciplines.

AMERICAN DENTAL HYGIENISTS ASSOCIATION (ADHA)

444 North Michigan Avenue
Suite 400
Chicago, IL 60611
(312) 440-8900
Website: www.adha.org
Facebook and Instagram: @youradha
The ADHA is a professional organization for dental hygienists. It provides educational information and career guidance.

BUREAU OF LABOR STATISTICS (BLS)

U.S. Department of Labor
Postal Square Building
2 Massachusetts Avenue NE
Washington, D.C. 20212-0001
(202) 691-5200
Website: www.bls.gov
The BLS is part of the Department of Labor. They publish facts and statistics about a multitude of careers.

CANADIAN DENTAL ASSOCIATION (CDA)

1815 Alta Vista Drive
Ottawa, ON K1G 3Y6
Canada
(613) 523-1770
Website: www.cda-adc.ca
Facebook: @CanadianDentalAssociation
Instagram: @cdndentalassoc
CDA is a professional organization for dentists practicing in Canada.

CANADIAN DENTAL HYGIENISTS ASSOCIATION (CDHA)

1122 Wellington Street, N.W.
Ottawa, ON K1Y 2Y7
Canada
(800) 267-5235 and (613) 224-5515
Website: www.cdha.ca
Facebook: @CDHAdentalhygienists
Instagram: @TheCDHA
The CDHA is a professional organization for dental hygienists practicing in Canada.

COMMISSION ON DENTAL ACCREDITATION (CODA)

211 East Chicago Avenue
Chicago, IL 60611
(800) 232-6108
Website: coda.ada.org
CODA is the organization within the ADA that accredits dental education programs in the US.

DR. SAMUEL D. HARRIS NATIONAL MUSEUM OF DENTISTRY

31 South Greene Street
Baltimore, MD 21201
(410) 706-0600
Website: www.dentalmuseum.com
Facebook and Instagram: @SDHNMD
The National Dental Museum is part of the Smithsonian, It's also associated with the University of Maryland School of Dentistry.

JOB CORPS

200 Constitution Avenue NW, Room N4459
Washington, D.C. 20210
(800) 733-JOBS [5627]
Website: www.jobcorps.gov
Facebook and Instagram: @DOLJobCorps
The Job Corps is Department of Labor program that provides free job training for young people. They offer a program to become a qualified dental assistant.

NATIONAL DENTAL HYGIENISTS ASSOCIATION (NDHA)

3060 Mitchellville Road
Suite 215
Bowie, MD 20716
(240) 241-4448
Website: ndaonline.org/national-dental-hygienists-assoc
The NDHA is a professional organization dedicated to promoting the interests of minority dental hygienists. It's associated with the National Dental Association.

FOR FURTHER READING

American Dental Association. *CDT 2023: Current Dental Terminology*. Chicago, IL: American Dental Association, 2023.

Cavazos, Tiffany. *HYGIENEPRENEUR*: *The Dental Hygienist's Guide to Achieving Career* Success & Personal *Transformation*. Independently published, 2021.

Dabas, Usha. *Dental Fundamentals for Auxiliary Staff: A Book For Dental Office Administrators*. Independently published, 2021.

Endsley, Kezia. *Dental Assistants and Hygienists: A Practical Career Guide*. Lanham, MD: Rowman & Littlefield, 2019.

Morkes, Andrew. *Dental Hygienists*. Chicago, IL: College and Career Press LLC, 2022.

Murray, Tamika. *Become a Dental Hygienist*. San Diego, CA: BrightPoint Press, 2023.

Samniczell Publication. *Dental Anatomy Coloring Book*. Independently published, 2020.

Sunspun Press. *So You Want to Be a Dental Assistant?* Independently published, 2023.

INDEX

ABOUT THE AUTHOR

KATHLEEN A. KLATTE is the author of many nonfiction books for children and teens. Topics range from animals and nature to constitutional law to unusual career choices. She lives in New York with one cat and far too many books and Legos.

PHOTO CREDITS

Photo credits: Cover, p. 1 R7 Photo/Shutterstock.com; Cover, pp. 1, 3-96 Merydolla/ Shutterstock.com; p. 4 Vasin Lee/Shutterstock.com; p. 5 DC Studio/Shutterstock.com; p. 7 weha/Shutterstock.com; p. 9 Ruslan Huzau/Shutterstock.com; p. 11 Teo Angelovski/ Shutterstock.com; pp. 13, 65, 74 Dragana Gordic/Shutterstock.com; p. 15 Avocado_studio/ Shutterstock.com; p. 17 InFocus.ee/Shutterstock.com; p. 19 Harbucks/Shutterstock. com; p. 21 Karkhut/Shutterstock.com; p. 23 AlessandroBiascioli/Shutterstock.com; p. 25 Evgeniy Kalinovskiy/Shutterstock.com; p. 27 LumenSt/Shutterstock.com; p. 29 xraytechnician/Shutterstock.com; p. 31 Sebastian Duda/Shutterstock.com; p. 33 rosco. shot/Shutterstock.com; p. 35 Pixel-Shot/Shutterstock.com; p. 36 al7/Shutterstock.com; p. 38 Ocskay Mark/Shutterstock.com; p. 39 Photoroyalty/Shutterstock.com; p. 41 https:// commons.wikimedia.org/wiki/File:J_S_Copley_-_Paul_Revere_(cropped).jpg; pp. 43, 45, 51, 69 Ground Picture/Shutterstock.com; p. 44 Drazen Zigic/Shutterstock.com; p. 47 Frame Stock Footage/Shutterstock.com; p. 49 CarlosBarquero/Shutterstock.com; p. 50 MakeStory Studio/Shutterstock.com; p. 52 FS Stock/Shutterstock.com; p. 53 KaryB/Shutterstock.com; p. 54 REDPIXEL.PL/Shutterstock.com; p. 55 8th.creator/ Shutterstock.com; p. 56 Monkey Business Images/Shutterstock.com; p. 57 New Africa/Shutterstock.com; p. 58 Bain News Service, Publisher. G. Washington's teeth. [Between and Ca. 1915] Photograph. Retrieved from the Library of Congress, <www. loc.gov/item/2014689477/>.; p. 59 Loveischiangrai/Shutterstock.com;p. 60 Roman Zaiets/Shutterstock.com; p. 61 gpointstudio/Shutterstock.com; p. 63 wavebreakmedia/ Shutterstock.com; p. 64 Svitlana Hulko/Shutterstock.com; p. 66 No-Te Eksarunchai/ Shutterstock.com; p. 67 Kravtzov/Shutterstock.com; p. 68 Oleksii Didok/Shutterstock. com; p. 70 baklykovadaria/Shutterstock.com; p. 71 kenchiro168/Shutterstock.com; p. 73 fizkes/Shutterstock.com; p. 75 bebebyul/Shutterstock.com; p. 77 https://commons. wikimedia.org/wiki/File:41D-03-027_-_STS-41D_-_STS-41D_crew_activities_-_ DPLA_-_7f01b11b230596278a5ede8279ae4336.jpg; p. 79 ADragan/Shutterstock.com; p. 80 fizkes/Shutterstock.com; p. 81 aodaodaodaod/Shutterstock.com; p. 82 bbernard/ Shutterstock.com.